PRISM

Shedding Light on
Life with Duchenne

by David K.

ISBN 978-1-7366463-0-4 (paperback)
ISBN 978-1-7366463-1-1 (ePub)
ISBN 978-1-7366463-2-8 (Kindle)

FOR PHILIP EDGERLEY

"THE HISTORICAL CONCEPTION OF DISEASE, THE IDEA THAT DISEASES HAVE A COURSE, FROM THEIR FIRST INTIMATIONS TO THEIR HAPPY OR FATAL RESOLUTION, TELLS US NOTHING ABOUT THE INDIVIDUAL, AND *HIS* HISTORY; CONVEYS NOTHING OF THE PERSON, AND THE EXPERIENCE OF THE PERSON, AS HE FACES, AND STRUGGLES TO SURVIVE HIS DISEASE."

Oliver Sacks

PROLOGUE

When I was young, my mom would hang these small golden animal figurines from the kitchen window, each with a small circular prism in the center. From my usual seat at the end of the kitchen table, I could see the dozens of tiny, oblong rainbows scattered about by the figurines. When I asked my mom why these rainbows would appear, she explained, "The prisms separate the light into all of its colors." This answer would not satisfy me for long.

I was soon interrogating my poor mother with even more questions: "Where do the colors come from?" "Why can't I see them?" "How can they be there if I can't see them?" As any good parent would do, she tried her best to nurture my curiosity by answering the questions in words I could understand.

My mom struggled to find the right words, and the best answer she could give was, "The colors are always there, you just can't see them." How could that be? The rainbows were invisible?! My five-year-old head was spinning. Something I thought I knew perfectly well—light, the most ordinary of phenomena—suddenly proved to be much more richly complex. I had assumed the light I could see with the naked eye, what I could see only at the surface, was all there is. Little did I know there was far more beauty and complexity to experience; I only had to look deeper.

Just like my five-year-old-self, most people don't even realize that their understanding of disability[1] is incomplete; they are entirely unaware of its richness hidden just slightly out of their view.

---

1 For the purposes of this book, any reference to disability will solely refer to individuals who use a wheelchair.

DISCLAIMER

This book is a memoir. It reflects the author's present recollections of the events described herein. All names and identifying information have been changed to protect the privacy of those mentioned, and some of the characters are composites of multiple individuals. Additionally, some events have been compressed, and the chronology has been slightly altered for narrative simplicity. Some dialogue has also been recreated.

INTRODUCTION

I was sitting in the lobby of the student union, with three of my friends, as we brainstormed ideas for our new blog. The blog, called *The Fine Scholars*, would detail our unique experiences as college students with severe disabilities.

We were all seniors, so we had plenty to talk about, from: our first taste of independence, to not knowing how to manage our own personal care, to our first beer.

It was really cool to look back on the previous five years, and see how much we had all changed.

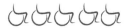

The conversation went on for hours, with a big focus on the Roberts program. This is the fully inclusive, fully adaptive residence hall that had allowed us to go away to school in the first place—all the unique experiences wouldn't have happened without it.

As we were wrapping things up, my friend Ron put it all in perspective: "Think about everything we've accomplished in the last five years: leaving the only caregivers we ever knew (our parents), learning how to train new caregivers, moving to a completely new place, learning to be independent—which is orders of magnitude more difficult for someone like us (someone with a severe disability) …" He continued ranting for a few minutes, and finally ended with: "*Oh yeah*, and on top of all of that, there's the 'small' matter of earning a college degree."

All I could say was, "Wow." I had to take a step back, and really think about where I was: "I use a power wheelchair. I can barely move my body. I use a machine to breathe. I need assistance with all of my daily care. Yet, here I am: about to graduate from a prestigious university."

As I reflected on my accomplishments, I almost couldn't believe they were real. I had to seriously ask myself: "How did I get here?"

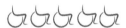

It's actually quite a tale: the story of how I "got there." And, luckily for you, it is the subject of the book you are about to read.

CHAPTER ONE

A GAME CHANGER

When I came into this world, there were no physical signs of a problem, no hints that something might be wrong. I cried, I opened my eyes and looked around. My mother held me lovingly, unaware of my preordained genetic destiny: a critical error hidden in my DNA.

My parents were spared this knowledge at first. In my early years, I learned to talk, I learned to walk; I met all the important milestones. I was happy. My parents were happy. We were all playing the usual game of life—the rules predictable, the challenges familiar. But inevitably, the game would change.

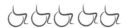

At the end of every summer, my grandparents would visit, and as grandparents do, they would spend as much time with my sister and me as possible. So naturally they wanted to go to my Little League tee-ball game.

All of the preschool-aged kids would run around in a disorganized mess and their parents called it a sport. Some bored kids would wander around the outfield while others were unsure of which direction to run on the base path. It was chaos, made cute by their aimlessness. Parents would swoon over their adorable kid in uniform, and my parents no doubt did the same. This affection likely distracted them from seeing that something was wrong.

My grandpa, who never shied away from speaking his mind and wasn't in the habit of sugar-coating anything, bluntly told my mom, "There's something wrong with him. He's running funny." Whether this was something my parents didn't see until then, or refused to believe they were seeing, no longer mattered. They saw it now.

I was quickly taken to the family doctor, who then referred us to a specialist. He sent my parents to a neurologist who in turn recommended a muscle biopsy.[2] The results came back. They were positive for something called Duchenne muscular dystrophy,[3] and the doctor had the unfortunate job of explaining to my parents what this condition would entail.

I still don't think I will ever grasp the emotional magnitude of hearing this news, and what it did to my parents. In an instant, everything changed. Several of the potential futures my parents may have imagined for me became impossibilities. I wouldn't be a sports star, a surgeon, or an airline pilot. Would I ever get married? Would I go to

---

2 A procedure where a small bit of tissue is extracted to analyze for diagnostic purposes.

3 Duchenne is a progressive condition characterized by increasing muscle weakness.

college? Would I even live long enough to be college-aged? The questions were endless.

My parents found themselves in this unforgiving wilderness with no idea how to survive. They were forced to wrestle with issues like health insurance, finding various specialist doctors, and keeping up to date with the latest medical literature. They had all these terms thrown at them: preventative medicine, palliative care, quality of life, and so on. They were in over their heads.

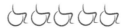

My experience of learning the news was vastly different. My parents told me that I had muscular dystrophy, and that was the extent of it.

The news didn't affect me in the least. As a five-year-old, I wasn't exactly future-oriented. I couldn't possibly understand the ways in which my condition would come to affect my life. All I knew was the here and now, and, at the moment, Duchenne didn't seem to affect my life in any way.[4] I knew I had a condition, but it became just another basic fact about myself that I could recite. As I knew my address and my phone number, I also knew the name of my disease.

---

4 The disease is progressive. That means the symptoms gradually get worse. At first, the effects are negligible.

CHAPTER TWO

THIS ISN'T SO BAD

PART ONE: SPECIAL TREATMENT

The first time my disability created any real problems was when I was in first or second grade. I was starting to experience some early symptoms: difficulty getting up off the ground, difficulty climbing stairs, difficulty walking long distances; and extra steps needed to be taken to ensure I could fully participate in school.

Since I went to St Benedict—a private, Catholic school, there were no strict guidelines on how to do this. My parents had to actually meet with school staff and brainstorm what academic accommodations I would need.[5]

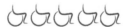

When my parents told me I would have to start doing certain things differently than my classmates, it was done in a gentle, reassuring way. But after I learned what my accommodations would be, I didn't need to be reassured;

---

5 The adjustments that allowed me to fully participate in a typical classroom at school. These included: changes to the arrangement of the classroom, the length of my bathroom breaks, and being excused from gym.

if anything, the whole situation seemed more like special treatment than something to be ashamed of.

When the entire class had to line up and march single file to the bathroom, I never had to go with them. The big student bathrooms were down three flights of stairs; it would take little David hours to make that trek. I was instead allowed "exclusive" access to the teacher's bathroom on the same level as my classroom. My disabled benefits package didn't end there. The school went to church once a week, and because I walked much slower than the other kids, I would leave early to walk to church and back. My favorite was gym class. I didn't have to go at all; I stayed in the classroom and played on the computer for an hour.

All of these little tweaks to my routine gave me a bit more freedom than the other kids. When I went to the teacher's bathroom, it was by myself. When I left to walk back and forth to church, I was by myself; and when I stayed back from gym, I was essentially by myself. The times spent unsupervised, by myself, are some of my fondest memories of grade school.

I'll admit, when my bathroom trips inevitably ended sooner, I didn't sit quietly at my desk, waiting for the class to return. For five minutes a day, there were no rules, and I took full advantage of it. I would go through the drawers in my teacher's desk. I would throw things out the open windows. I might have "borrowed" school supplies from my classmates' desks. The best part was, no one ever knew about it.

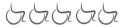

Due to the constant games of tag and football, recess was eventually added to the list of times where I wouldn't participate with everyone else. However, I wouldn't be completely alone; five minutes is one thing, leaving me by myself for the entire fifteen minutes of recess was not going to happen. My mom spoke with the school and requested that one of my friends be allowed to stay inside with me during recess. My mom would know I was getting some social time during recess, and she wouldn't have to worry that I was by myself for so long.

Having a friend with me may have been safer, but it certainly didn't stop me from enjoying my unsupervised time. If anything, I became bolder now that I had an accomplice. After lunch, my friend James and I would head back to the classroom, and the shenanigans would begin.

One of my favorite things to do was flick paper footballs. With no one around, we could really get some distance on those things. This then evolved into what we liked to call "catapulting," in which you place a pen or pencil on the edge of a desk and hit it as hard as you can with a ruler. This didn't last long. Catapulting came to an abrupt end after we got several pens stuck inside the ceiling lights.

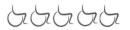

THIS ISN'T SO BAD

PART TWO: BEING CREATIVE

As with the paper footballs and pens, I always seemed to find alternatives to the typical physically-focused games that boys played.

When the weather was warm, kids wanted to play outside. This often meant riding one of a variety of vehicles, whether it be bikes, Big Wheels, scooters, or wagons. I couldn't keep up on my mobility scooter. I didn't have the horsepower. What I would often do instead was offer to be their "rickshaw driver." We would tie our wagon to the back of my scooter, and I would drag my friends around.

As time went on, I got more inventive, and the stunts became more dangerous. My cousin Luke had a Razor Scooter, to which we attached a bungee cord. It worked pretty well, but we realized it was too short. So, we attached three more bungee cords to the first one. We rambled down the street, neither of us having any real way to control our creation. During our very first test run, I took a very wide turn on to the cross street and Luke, tethered to eight feet of bungee cords, took a much wider turn. He slammed head-on into a parked car. We tried one more time, and the bungee cord snapped and hit me right in the ass. The bungee cord was retired shortly after.

My friend James and I had a novel method for using my old wagon. He would sit in the wagon, holding the handle to steer, and I would push from behind. After mastering the art of coordinated driving, we would cruise up and down the block at a respectable speed.

We never really had any incidents, except one. The wagon veered off course and was heading toward a very big, muddy, puddle at the end of the alley. James jumped out to avoid ending up face-first in the mud, but instead collided with my motorized scooter at full speed. After he smacked into the ground, I couldn't stop and ended up running over his arm. We were both lucky it wasn't broken.

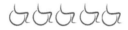

THIS ISN'T SO BAD

PART THREE: MAKE MY WISH COME TRUE

One day, completely out of the blue, my dad tells me something mind-blowing: "There is an organization called the Make-A-Wish foundation. They give wishes to disabled kids, and you're eligible. You can have whatever wish you want!" I immediately pictured the genie from *Aladdin*, granting three wishes. I assumed that my dad was joking: "Whatever, dad!"

My mom stepped in: "No David, it's the truth." It was the pre-internet days, so my dad physically handed me the paper brochure that had come in the mail. I saw several pictures of other kids on their wishes. One kid was pictured with Michael Jordan, another with an entire room full of toys. The excitement was building. "I can wish to meet Michael Jordan? I can wish for a shopping spree at Toys 'R' Us?!" My dad interjected, "You can wish for anything you want..."

My mind was racing with possibilities. How was I supposed to decide? In the mail, we had also gotten a form for me to fill out. It was a two-by-two grid, and I was supposed to draw four different things that I would like to wish for, in order of preference. It took several weeks of conversations with my parents and a ton of brainstorming to come up with my four choices.

My first choice was by far the most creative: go to Hawaii and fly over an erupting volcano. The second choice was to meet Jim Carrey, as I was obsessed with the movies *Ace Ventura: Pet Detective* and *Liar Liar*, this was followed by a shopping spree and a go-cart. The volcano thing was deemed too dangerous, so I ended up with my second choice of meeting Jim Carrey.

The next step was an in-home meeting with some Make-A-Wish people. We were briefed on all the details of the wish. The four of us would fly out to California and stay for a week. Each day seemed more awesome than the next. The first two days we were free to explore Hollywood. One day I would receive the VIP treatment at Universal Studios. The next day I had my choice of VIP treatment at either Disneyland or Knott's Berry Farm (like Disneyland but with Peanuts characters). The week would culminate in a private dinner with Jim Carrey—private enough, at least; there would be four or five other kids and their families meeting with him as well. I could barely think straight at the prospect of how amazing it all sounded.

The trip would be in early October. It was currently April. I didn't know how I would be able to wait six months. The wait was agonizing; it was worse than waiting for Christmas.

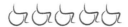

The morning of our departure, my family and I were waiting to be picked up. Make-A-Wish would be taking care of all transportation, from beginning to end. To my surprise, the driver did not show up in a van or a taxi but in a giant stretch limousine. Even my parents seemed surprised.

The driver and my dad put our bags in the trunk, and we all got settled. It turned out that the transportation was ahead of schedule and there was some time to kill, and I got to decide how the extra time would be spent. Since it was a regular weekday, right around the time the neighborhood kids were walking to school, I wanted to go pick up my friends and drop them off at school.

My neighborhood is relatively small, so we had enough time to swing by and pick up several of my classmates, and even a few older kids my parents knew. The inside of that limo was crammed to capacity with neighborhood kids: Kenny, Robert, Mary, and James. All of us felt pretty cool pulling up in front of school in a limousine.

Soon after chauffeuring my friends to school, the time for showing off was over; we headed for the airport. It was my first time on an airplane, which was exciting in itself for a seven-year-old boy, but it was made better by the fact that we flew first class. A stewardess brought us ice cream and orange soda. Another stewardess brought my sister and I search-and-find puzzles similar to "Where's Waldo?" After four hours, we arrived and were greeted at the airport by two Make-A-Wish representatives, who had gifts for my sister and me: model toy cars. It would seem someone at the office made a mistake in remembering the gender of my sibling, but could we really complain?

Over the next few days, the four of us had a blast at Universal Studios and Knott's Berry Farm, enjoying my VIP treatment at each. We also enjoyed the Hollywood Walk of Fame and Venice Beach. Then, at long last, it was the big day. All of the families were to be picked up by a tram from the Universal Studios Backlot Tour ride, driven to the park, and given the tour, with the last stop being a specially reserved Italian restaurant.

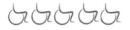

The families were seated at two or three different tables. There was a buffet of artisan pizzas, breadsticks, and pasta and a palpable sense of anticipation. We were briefed by some stiff in a suit about the procedure: "Mr. Carrey will visit with each child in order from the front of the room to the back of the room. Each child is allotted exactly fifteen minutes with Mr. Carrey." This went on for several minutes, but none of us really took that woman seriously. After the robotic bureaucrat was done talking, the man of the hour casually entered the room with a big smile.

The room naturally went nuts with applause. The same emotionless woman interrupted this elation and directed him toward the first table. I was at the second table, beginning to freak out. He eventually came to our table and sat right next to me. I couldn't say a word. I was in awe. Here he was, the real guy, Ace Ventura himself, and not on the TV, but in real life. He was actually a real person just like me! I wasted most of my "allotted" time awkwardly laughing and tripping over my words. There were plenty of things I had planned to say to him, but my mind was a blank.

Only after Jim left to visit with the other girl across the table was my mind flooded with all of my previously forgotten questions. I was feeling like I had wasted my chance, but once I saw how prepared this other girl was, it really sunk in how much more I could have done. She pulled out a tape recorder and began recording their conversation.

Then, her dad showed up with a giant cardboard cut-out of Jim Carrey from one of those movie theater promotional things—from the movie *Liar Liar* by the looks of it. He was asked to autograph his likeness and, in classic Jim Carrey fashion, proceeded to draw a mustache on the face and color in one of the teeth. At that point, I just had to give her props. She was doing the Make-A-Wish thing right.

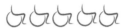

Before I knew it, the dinner was over. I was still in shock that I got to meet "the funniest man alive." The next day we would be heading to the airport to return home, and though I was disappointed my trip was coming to an end, I was still happy. Unprepared or not, I got to meet my hero.

We flew home, again in first class. We were given a ride home, again in a limo. After all was said and done, the only thing I could say was, "Wow!"

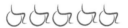

Several years after being diagnosed, having muscular dystrophy still didn't seem that bad. There were a few symptoms I had to deal with, but they were nothing more than an inconvenience. To me, the good far outweighed the bad. After all, I was able to skip gym and use a private bathroom. I even got to meet Jim Carrey. As far as I was concerned, everything was just fine.

However, this ignorant bliss wouldn't last forever. The novelty of accommodations, and of being different in general, would quickly wear off.

CHAPTER THREE

NOT ALL SUNSHINE AND RAINBOWS

PART ONE: WELL, THIS IS EMBARRASSING

With each passing year, the level of accommodations I needed increased. Quite inconveniently, the increase in accommodations happened around the same time I began to care about what people thought of me.

My mom got a job as the lunch lady at my school, which enabled her to help me during her breaks. This was, of course, the only option to allow me to stay at the same school. But I didn't think about it that way. All I knew was the assistance from my mom occurred in plain sight and elicited gawking and staring from my peers.

My classmates eventually became desensitized to the sight of an eleven-year-old kid being carried around piggyback-style by his mother, but anyone else would stare blankly. My mom would carry me to my seat in the morning, and it was fine. My friends would say "Hi" to me and "Hi, Mrs. K." to my mom. This occurred every day; it was no big deal. But, if my mom carried me to the lunchroom or the auditorium, kids from other classes would be amazed.

Once a week, my fourth-grade class would go to the preschool classroom. We had a mentoring-type arrangement with them; our two classes would get together and do a craft or something. The preschool class was on the opposite side of the building, one floor below. This was quite the trek for my mom, who had to carry me the entire way on her back.

One week in particular, my class had to wait outside for a few minutes, as the preschool class had not returned from the bathroom. The whole class waited in single file, with my mom and me at the back of the line. As we were standing there, another class returned from the bathroom and waited directly across from us for their door to be unlocked. I felt the immediate burn of forty little eyes aimed in my direction. It was the look I was becoming accustomed to, and yet was still entirely uncomfortable with—that gaping, wide-mouthed, bewildered look. I tried to ignore it and look away, but my face became flushed hot.

We probably only spent a minute or two waiting outside the preschool door, but it felt like hours. This was one of the first times I remember feeling acutely self-aware of my disability, and it wouldn't be the last.

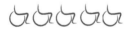

NOT ALL SUNSHINE AND RAINBOWS

PART TWO: RIDING THE BENCH

I grew up in the nineties, so I loved the Chicago Bulls. I had multiple Michael Jordan jerseys and hundreds of hours clocked in for *NBA Shootout 2001* on the PlayStation One. I was also involved with my school's basketball team as much as I could be. Whoever the coaches were, they always made an effort to include me. I was allowed to sit on the bench with the team and keep stats on every player. I had my own jersey, and I even got a trophy when the team won the Catholic League Championship.

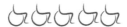

Eventually we found a way for me to play, by getting a basketball net next to the pool in the backyard. Playing with my friends, sister and dad, I was able to participate because we adjusted the rules a little. Whenever I got the ball close to the basket, the action stopped, my dad would toss me in the air, and I would basically slam dunk. My sister, and whichever friend was over, understood that the rules needed to be different for me and always graciously allowed my automatic points.

Then, one night, the inevitable happened; my physical limitations clashed with my love of a purely physical game. I was in the pool with three friends, and my dad wasn't there. So, when the game started, there was no one to enforce the inclusive rules. For a while, they cooperated and allowed me to take uncontested shots. But, being eleven-year-old boys, they got carried away and amped up the intensity. I knew I couldn't keep up so I backed off. I tried shouting comments to stay involved: "Air Ball!" "Nice shot!" However, my comments were given little acknowledgment in lieu of the action. For the first time, I strongly yearned to play basketball for real.

Later that night, I remember breaking down in tears, "I hate basketball! I hate sports! What's the point of caring about sports if I can't play them?!" I cried in my dad's arms, and he kept saying, "I know, I know. It sucks." What else could he say?

When football began shortly after, I was offered a similar "assistant coach" role with that team. I refused it. From my point of view, it was just some hollow position created to include me. I didn't want to be included; I wanted to actually play.

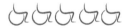

NOT ALL SUNSHINE AND RAINBOWS

PART THREE: MAKING SENSE OF THINGS

I was starting to notice a pattern in the way other people were treating me. I began to receive a lot of undeserved attention; acquaintances were being extremely nice, too nice, to the point where it seemed patronizing. I would simply take a walk[6] in the neighborhood, and you would think I was a damn celebrity: everyone was thrilled to see me. It was like people got excited when they had a sighting of "the wheelchair boy."

I suppose it's easy to remember the name of the kid in the wheelchair. But, on my end, it was a little more difficult. I would be greeted by friends of friends, people I may have only met once, people I vaguely recognized but had never spoken to, and adults in the neighborhood whose names I couldn't have been expected to know. It was the ultimate nightmare scenario: that interaction where someone familiar knows your name but you don't remember theirs; and it was happening several times a week.

At first, I tried my best to be polite to everyone and fulfill my social responsibilities. But there was so much attention being thrown at me, that it was starting to become a chore to deal with.

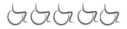

After a while, I was burned out. I only had so much energy for small talk and social etiquette. I eventually started ignoring it. Someone would shout out my name from behind or from across the street, and instead of identifying who it

---

6 Just a phrase. "Taking a walk," is easier to say than "taking a ride in my wheelchair."

was and shouting back to them, I ignored it. The parent of a random schoolmate would try to talk to me, and I would answer their initial question and simply keep going. On several occasions, I even blatantly ignored people, cruising right on past without saying anything. I started to get a reputation as rude from my classmates and neighbors.

As much as neighbors talk, my behavior eventually came to the attention of my parents, and I was given the typical parental "talking to." But I didn't change. I remember one incident very clearly. My class had taken a field trip to the local museum, and my dad was necessarily a chaperone—as usual. Out of the entire class, a random couple singled me out—I wonder why—to speak to, and I didn't want any part of it. My dad corrected me on the spot. The couple, lending assistance to my dad in parenting added, "Your dad is right, not talking to people is rude."

I was trapped in quite the double bind. On one hand, I didn't like being patronized, and on the other hand I was told that ignoring the unwanted attention was unacceptable. I had to oblige the unwarranted kindness or face social punishment by being labeled rude.

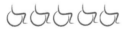

I was in early adolescence, still beginning to form my identity. This would be difficult enough for anyone, but I had the added task of trying to understand how disability fit into the equation.

Were people being overly nice because I was disabled or was it something specific to me that invited this weird treatment? I would soon have my answer. We had a neighbor with spina bifida, Carl, an older man in a manual wheelchair.[7] He would often sit outside and listen to baseball games on the radio. Being the close-knit community that it was, many neighbors and acquaintances would stop by and chat with him—and they would talk with him with kid gloves. Imagine teenagers and twenty-somethings calling a sixty-year-old man buddy as in, "Hey buddy what's the score of the game?" I recall my dad once asking Carl how the Cubs did that day, even though he had already watched the game. I asked my dad why he had done that, and his answer was, "You'll understand when you're older."

Ok, so people were overly nice to people with disabilities. My next question was, "Why?" After watching a video in health class, I had my answer to that question as well. It was the same tired "drinking is bad" message I had been bombarded by for years. The narrator began with something cheesy like "John and Sally thought having a few drinks would be innocent fun. BUT THEN…" After several minutes of a completely inauthentic re-creation of teenage drinking, the video got to the point: "It was time to head home, and John thought he would be okay to drive." Then things got serious as the real "Sally" came on screen to describe what happened next. She was paralyzed in the accident and in a wheelchair, speaking with one of those

---

7 A wheelchair that is self-propelled. It can also be pushed by others.

computer boxes. She started to say things like "You don't want to end up like me."

Was having a disability going to be like that when I got older? Absolutely horrible? No hope? Maybe that was why people were overly nice, because they felt bad, because they knew what was coming.

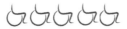

Without even understanding what was happening, I was already beginning to succumb to the pressure and conform to that "sympathetic charity-case" role. I was getting all this feedback from the media, neighbors, and even trusted adults. What other conclusion was I going to make?

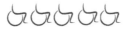

NOT ALL SUNSHINE AND RAINBOWS

PART FOUR: AN UNFORTUNATE ACCIDENT

I had just finished sixth grade and was looking forward to the summer ahead. But, before summer vacation really picked up, I had one major obligation—my sister's annual dance recital. I always hated going to those. We were there to see Liz's dance class perform their routine. I didn't care about the twenty other routines I was made to sit through. My perfectly logical argument, that we should leave after my sister's performance, always fell on deaf ears: "You can't leave, that's rude." But, this year, surprisingly, I was allowed to stay at my friend James's house.

I was relieved and gladly rode my motorized scooter to James's house on the next block. I entered through the backyard, via the alley, as usual, James opening the back gate. I pulled up to the back porch and was met by my dad, dressed in a shirt and tie; he had come to carry me up the stairs before heading to the recital. He set me down on a rolling office chair; I didn't have my manual wheelchair, so this would have to suffice for the night.

It was a fun time; we played several hours of *Grand Theft Auto III* on PlayStation 2 and looked at pictures of naked ladies on the computer. The entire evening passed relatively quickly and before I knew it, my dad returned to carry me back down the stairs to my scooter still parked outside. He scooped me up and headed toward the door. We were about to go down the stairs, and then suddenly we were both on the ground. My dad must have had bad footing or something because we only made it down one stair before tumbling down the other three.

Immediately, I had an intense aching pain in my right leg. James's mom gave me some Tylenol and I laid on their couch for a while. After nothing changed for a half-hour, my dad decided I should get an x-ray. He called an ambulance, as being transported by stretcher would be gentler on my potentially broken leg than being carried.

After spending a few hours in the emergency room, I

was given an x-ray, and indeed my femur had a slight break above the right knee. Luckily, I wouldn't need surgery, but I would have to get a cast.

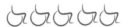

Being in a cast for eight weeks would certainly change my summer plans—a change I was not pleased about to say the least. I wasn't able to go swimming or ride around the neighborhood in my shiny, new power wheelchair every day. This was especially unfortunate because I had just recently been allowed to freely traverse the neighborhood, crossing the street by myself and coming and going as I pleased. Instead of exploring my new freedom, I would have to remain in bed with my leg elevated.

I made my unhappiness known, and my mom had to set me straight: "It sucks, but there's nothing you can do about it. You might as well make the best of it." I begrudgingly agreed to try.

We got one of those heavy armchair pillows made specifically for sitting against and a "breakfast-in-bed" tray on which I could keep the remote and the PS2 controller. It was not a bad setup. On top of that, my friends Robert and John began coming over semi-regularly to play video games. It would seem I wasn't going to have a hard time keeping busy.

For the first few weeks it was great. I sat in my bed all day, even eating meals on my bed tray. My uncle would bring over whatever junk food I asked for—Little Caesars, White Castle, ice cream. My dad felt bad and offered to buy me a Game Boy Advance, an awesome apology gift if there is such a thing. I had never binged so hard on video games or anime, and friends seemed to come over even more than before.

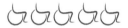

It was only a matter of time until weeks of bed rest got old. Soon the initial "emergency response" from everyone subsided and the extra attention ceased. All I was left with was an intense feeling of boredom. Sure, my uncle was still coming over once in a while, and my friends would still come to play video games, but I spent the majority of the time by myself in my room.

It didn't happen consciously, but I started to seek out things to distract myself. I found my obsession in the *Madden* football video game. I would get up in the morning and turn it on, playing continuously until I went to sleep. One game would end, and I would immediately start another one. The obsession was fierce, and eventually my self-esteem became entirely contingent upon my *Madden* performance each day. If I were to lose a lot, my family would suffer my wrath.

This went on for weeks. I did perfect my skills, but I had no one to show them off to. It was a hollow feeling. Video games were no longer enough to distract myself. The only

25

thing that would cure my boredom was getting the cast off. I needed to get in the pool, to feel the warmth of the sun on my face. I needed to join the kids I could hear playing through the window.

My whole family was ready for my cast to come off, so much so that my dad cut it off himself with a hand saw. It was time for my hermit-like existence to come to an end.

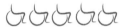

The first chance I got, I went out to see what my friends were up to. I came across a big herd of migrating preteens and was excited upon recognizing it as a group of my classmates: James, John, Robert, Kenny, Mary, and the other girls. They were happy to see me, as I had not been out in the neighborhood since I had broken my leg. I was equally excited to see them, but something felt strange.

My interactions didn't happen automatically. I found myself consciously planning out what to say and second-guessing myself. This had never happened before and caught me off guard. Later that night I was preoccupied, trying to figure out what had happened. I concluded that all my solitude during the summer must have made me a little rusty at talking to people.

Then, another awkward experience rattled my confidence even more. It was my friend Robert's Memorial Day barbecue, and all the kids my age were setting off fireworks in the empty lot behind the house. As I approached,

I could hear them naïvely talking about sex, as adolescent kids tend to do. When I got there, the girl who was speaking stopped midsentence as if she could no longer discuss mature topics in front of someone in a wheelchair.

I immediately picked up on her reaction, but apparently no one else had. I saw Robert's face, and then I looked at my friend Kenny's. They didn't seem to realize I was being treated differently. Being the only one to notice, I started to doubt that I was being treated differently because I was disabled; maybe I was just acting awkwardly. I honestly didn't know.

I started to worry I had lost it, lost the ability to socialize properly. Could a few weeks of bed rest have done that much damage? It's not like I was completely alone the entire time. Deep down I knew it was irrational and tried to convince myself to snap out of it. "You can't just forget how to talk to people. That's not how that works." As much sense as my inner dialogue made, and as much as I was aware that the whole thing was silly, my social woes continued.

After a few weeks of mild awkwardness, I had an experience that was much more intense, genuine social anxiety. I remember passing by my school and seeing Robert and a few others as I passed; they were unloading some boxes, helping prepare for Market Day.[8] I was greeted and prompted with conversation. All I could muster was a "Hi," and didn't even slow down as I continued past. I could

---

8 A weekly discounted grocery-delivery service.

hear a voice saying, "Wait, come back for a second," but I was too overcome with anxiety to stop. My mind became laser-focused on getting home. The safety of my bedroom was just minutes away, and that's all I could think of.

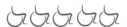

After this most recent incident, I said, "Enough is enough. I am not going to be afraid of people!" I forced myself to go out to the neighborhood hangout—the park—and see what would happen if I pushed through and endured the panic. I can still vividly remember that day; I could literally feel myself trembling with fear. My friends tried to talk to me, but all I could manage were one- or two-word responses. Then, I sat and watched a few of the guys play basketball at an unnecessarily far distance.

After a while, the anxiety built up and I went home. I asked my mom to transfer me to my bed, and she asked, "What's wrong? You look like you are going to cry." I said I was fine and just needed to lie down.

After I calmed down and composed myself, I was faced with a decision. Did I go back out and face this or give up and succumb to fear? Then—no joke—Phil Collins's song *Look Through My Eyes* from the Disney movie *Brother Bear* played on the TV. One of the lyrics goes like this: "There will be times on this journey when all you see is darkness. But somewhere out there, daylight finds you if you keep believing." As cheesy as that song is, it inspired me to get up and go back out. I got back in my wheelchair and set out to conquer my fears.

Upon seeing my friends again, everything was fine. I wasn't sure what had fixed the problem, but the anxiety seemed to be gone. I wasn't second-guessing myself, and I didn't feel that acute sense of fear anymore. I guess the moral of the story is to listen to a Disney song when you need motivation; that shit works!

CHAPTER FOUR

A COMMUNITY COMES TOGETHER

No matter the difficulties I faced, they always seemed to be dwarfed by the support my family and I received from the community. Our neighbors, family, and friends never missed an opportunity to lend a hand. Whether it be including me on the basketball team or the school allowing me and a friend to stay in the classroom during recess, we never felt alone to deal with the situation.

ᎶᎶᎶᎶᎶ

A COMMUNITY COMES TOGETHER

PART ONE: THE SCHOOL SITUATION

As mentioned previously, I went to a private, Catholic school—St. Benedict; they weren't necessarily equipped to handle a student with a disability, and my accommodations were consequently informal and somewhat improvised. On top of that, there were no government mandates for accessibility, no government mandates to accept someone like me as a student, and no government funding to provide any support services like occupational therapy or personal care aides. With no significant funding, the facilities were also outdated and barely adequate for someone like me—there wasn't even an elevator.

Despite all these shortcomings, I completed my entire elementary education and middle school, K–8, with no significant issues. I barely noticed any limitations in what the school could provide, given a little cooperation and generosity from the St. Benedict community.

To begin with, the mere fact I was able to continue to attend the school was a result of outside intervention. The principal, Mr. Gordon, had intended to leave around my fifth or sixth grade year. This would have endangered my ability to attend St. Benedict; there was no telling how the replacement principal would react to me and my improvised accommodations. A new person might decide it was a liability for me to stay. None of these potential consequences were even considered by my parents, as they had no way of knowing that Mr. Gordon intended to leave.

Unbeknownst to us, my aunt, who was a teacher at the school, pleaded with him to stay until I finished eighth grade. He agreed and stayed three extra years, leaving the very next year after I had left.

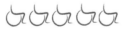

My mother's job as the lunch lady allowed her to help me

at school whenever I needed it, except, not surprisingly, during lunch. For a while, I was able to make it to the cafeteria on my own, but it soon became ridiculously impractical for me to do so. We needed a solution to get me back and forth to lunch.

My cousin Eric, who was several years older than me—he was in eighth grade when I was in third—volunteered to help carry me up and down the stairs to lunch. It probably wasn't that big of a sacrifice for him, seeing as he got to leave class early for lunch and return late to class after lunch, but it was a tremendous help to us.

Every day Eric would arrive about ten minutes before lunch, scoop me up piggyback- style, and trot down the several flights of stairs to the cafeteria. Then, he would come get me after lunch and take me back to my class. Eric and I would even sometimes race my friend[9] up the stairs if the coast was clear.

After Eric finished eighth grade and moved on to high school, another eighth-grader, our neighbor Jose, would provide my transportation for the year. And it would have been nice to continue this pattern of having an eighth grader help me each year, but it wasn't sustainable. I eventually became too big for a kid to carry.

My mom asked Mr. Johnson, one of the volunteer lunchroom aides, if he would be willing to do it, and he agreed. This would end up being a better solution, as he <u>was a grown man and could</u> easily carry me.

9 Recall, from chapter two that I always had a friend to stay inside with me during recess.

ᘒᘒᘒᘒᘒ

After a few more years, even having a grown man carry me up and down the stairs started to become impractical. I was just too big to be carried that far, down that many stairs. What were my parents going to do then? They were sort of out of options at that point.

The difficult decision was made for me to begin attending a public school. I would have to leave St. Benedict, the only school I had ever known, and attend Lincoln School. It was apparently the most disability-friendly public school in our area. But I didn't care about that. I would be leaving all my friends, leaving the familiarity of a school I had attended for five years. I wasn't thrilled.

ᘒᘒᘒᘒᘒ

It was a very strange experience: going to a new school—a lot of new experiences for me. The first day, I was picked up by the school bus—I'd never ridden one before. I had to push my own manual wheelchair all day—I wasn't physically prepared for that. The woman who helped secure my wheelchair in the bus and the woman who helped me use the bathroom were complete strangers—I wasn't too comfortable with that. The list goes on.

I wasn't bothered by most of these new experiences, but one thing in particular immediately turned me off to

Lincoln School. The environment at Lincoln was cold and impersonal. St. Benedict had a warm, small-town feel. Everything was personal and informal. I lived within walking distance of every one of my classmates, and I was often greeted by parents dropping off classmates. I personally knew the people assisting me: my mom helped me use the bathroom, a familiar lunchroom volunteer carried me to the lunchroom and got my food, and I knew the other staff members by name. At Lincoln, I knew no one.

In the formal, regimented system of accommodations, I often felt like I was on an assembly line, assisted and immediately passed down. On the first day, my very first interaction with a staff member was being pushed in my manual wheelchair from the bus to a long hallway just inside the door. Hardly any words were spoken as I was left in the hallway and told to wait until the bell rang. Seeing all the other wheelchair-using students slowly brought into the same hallway reminded me of herding cattle.

Lunch had the same vibe. The girl that helped get my food didn't even ask where I wanted to sit, leaving me at the first open table. I had to wheel myself to the table with my classmates.

My first experience with a personal-care aide wasn't any different. I went to the bathroom, and the girl grabbed this odd-looking metal container, from a shelf above the sinks, and proceeded to untie my pants. I asked what was going on, and she replied, "This is the spare urinal. You will have to use this since you don't have your own." I had never encountered a "urinal" before, though I immediately deduced what the small container was for.

It grossed me out to put my junk anywhere near a spare urinal that several people had probably used. I quickly asked where mine was and the aide replied as she pointed to the same shelf, which also had several plastic urinals, with names written on them in black marker, "You will have to bring yours from home like they did."

I agreed to get my own urinal, but I flat-out refused to use the spare one. I wasn't going near that germ factory, and insisted I use the toilet. The girl agreed, though not without attitude, to help get me on the toilet. I had never given instructions to anyone on how to help me, so I didn't say anything. I let this girl figure it out. She held me up with one arm and struggled to get my pants down with the other arm; it was a race to finish as I was slowly drooping toward the floor. I eventually made it onto the toilet, did my business, and left the bathroom unharmed, but I didn't like to be told how to use the bathroom. From then on, I used a different bathroom, and struggled to climb on and off the toilet by myself.

After the first day, I knew I didn't want to stay at that school. I pleaded my case to my mom when I got home. She wanted me to at least give it a chance, but my mind was made up. I pleaded every day for two weeks and she finally relented: "Okay I will get the transfer process started, but you are going to Lincoln until the paperwork goes through." Now there was an end in sight, and all I had to do was last a few more weeks.

One afternoon in mid-October, I disembarked from the school bus and headed toward the back door. I was busy contemplating my homework for the evening when my mom told me she had some good news. The transfer papers had gone through, and I would be returning to St. Benedict the very next day.

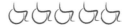

A COMMUNITY COMES TOGETHER

PART TWO: THE BUILD

As soon as I was greeted by name by the librarian, I knew I was where I was supposed to be. I was happy to be back, and my parents were happy I was back. But that didn't change the fact there was still no real solution for getting me up and down the stairs. Mr. Johnson was too nice to refuse to carry me, but it was clear the task wasn't easy for him. My parents would have to find another solution, but where to begin?

Upon learning of our dilemma, two women from the neighborhood took it upon themselves to organize a fundraiser to build some ramps. The ramps would lead into the main entrance of the school, and presumably allow me access to the lunchroom and my classroom as well.

The fundraiser was not just a bake sale or something to raise a few hundred dollars; it was going to be a huge block party with a goal in the tens of thousands. People would pay to eat and drink, and there would also be raffle tickets and other fundraisers.

I was too young to understand that my ability to attend St. Benedict was in question, or to appreciate this outpouring of support from the neighborhood. All I knew was there was a party being thrown just for me.

I was excited to be the guest of honor, though my parents had more to be concerned with. They didn't want to seem ungrateful or disrespectful with all the kindness and attention, and they scrambled to decide on the most respectful and socially acceptable response. Did they show up at the very beginning or wait a few hours? Did they spend the entire time thanking everybody? There wasn't exactly a precedent for how to act when having a massive benefit organized on behalf of your son.

We ended up going to the benefit a few hours after it began, my dad explaining, "It wouldn't be proper to show up right at the beginning." When we finally arrived, several people asked me where I had been, so who knows what the "best" response was. Either way, to me, it just seemed like any other summer block party. I ate the food and played with the other kids.

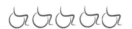

The fundraiser was such a success that my dad and my friend James's dad, Mr. Wilson, began throwing around the idea of building an elevator instead. This would be an ideal solution, but a far greater undertaking than simply building some ramps. There would be: planning, construction, permits, labor, someone to coordinate everything; and on top of all of that, construction would have to be entirely finished during the summer, before school started again.

To everyone's surprise, the job quickly became far less daunting. It would seem, they had underestimated the limits of the local people's generosity. My dad went to see an architect, to have them draw up the plans. Upon learning what the plans were for, there was no charge. There were negotiations with an elevator salesman, who, upon learning what the elevator would be for, gave them a huge discount. When it came to the actual construction, my family members and neighbors worked as volunteers. And, as fate would have it, my dad had been working for a construction equipment rental company for several years. My dad asked to rent some of the equipment, and upon learning what it was for, there was no charge.

According to the architect, a project of that magnitude would normally cost around $250,000 when taking into account equipment and labor; my dad and a few neighbors did it with less than one sixth of that.

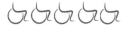

After three months, there was now an elevator where there wasn't before. When school started in the fall, the elevator took its maiden voyage. Instead of being carried up the stairs, I was able to climb the three stories and enter my classroom without ever leaving my wheelchair.

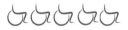

A COMMUNITY COMES TOGETHER

PART THREE: NOT TO BE DENIED

In my youth, when it came to typical social experiences, I was not deprived. My friends James and Robert were avid gamers like myself, and they were always over playing. I was also never at a loss for friends to share in my various fixations, whether it was Scooby-Doo, Power Rangers, or Pokémon. In particular, my friend Kenny and I shared a strong passion for Dragon Ball Z. We would count down the days until new episodes premièred, and together we were slowly amassing a giant collection of action figures—which we actually played with; none of that "never take it out of the box," collector shit.

Childhood experiences that would seem especially difficult to provide to someone like me, were also never out of reach. I went over to friends' houses; my dad or one of my friends' parents would carry me up the stairs. I spent the night at friends' houses, my friends often helping reposition me at night.

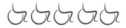

On a few rare occasions, I was even able to go away for the weekend with a friend's family. Kenny's parents had a cottage in Wisconsin, and one fall, my family was invited to spend the weekend. There were several families invited, so the fact I *needed* my parents there to help me was not a concern; I wouldn't be the only one with my parents there.

I was filled with anticipation during the three-hour drive, partly because I didn't do things like that very often, but mostly for the fall festivities. When we arrived at the house, my motorized scooter was left outside, covered with a tarp. The first night was spent playing board games and watching movies, and in the morning, we prepared for a long day.

All the festivities—a fair, a pumpkin patch, an apple orchard, a haunted house, etc.—were hosted at a fall-themed market-type complex. When we first pulled up to the place, I wasn't sure how I was going to get around—the ground was all mud, with a few patches of dead grass—but, everything worked out; the adults made sure I wasn't left out of anything. If my scooter got stuck in the grass, my dad was there to push it out. When I couldn't climb up into the hayride trailer, my dad and another dad lifted me. And, when the hedge maze, made of old corn stalks, was too narrow for my scooter, I forced my way in; I may have destroyed a lot of corn stalks and gotten scratched up a little, but it was worth it.

The next day was spent relaxing, hanging out, and enjoying the fall weather. Kenny, his brother and cousin, and I went down to the "beach," which was basically a small patch of land, next to a tiny lake, with dirt instead of sand. There was also a playground with an old rusted swing set and weeds growing up through the asphalt; it looked like those pictures of the abandoned city next to Chernobyl. I wasn't too keen on sticking around, so I headed back to the house.

To my dismay, the kids and some of the dads were playing tag football in the yard. I was not about to feel left out and decided to turn around. I began to head back to the Chernobyl park when my dad asked, "Where are you going?!" The group seemed determined to include me so I reluctantly agreed. The game was surprisingly enjoyable even though they ran noticeably slower when I had the ball, and let me score an obviously contrived touchdown.

Everything was going well until one particular play where my dad teasingly rushed at me full speed. It was clear he had intended to stop before he got to me, but he must have lost his balance because he ended up colliding with me. I was full-on tackled, scooter and all. The scooter tipped over, and I took a significant portion of my dad's weight. If not for the armrest on my scooter chair acting as a shield, I would've taken the full force of my dad's tackle.

Luckily, I was not hurt, and I managed to not get tackled again the rest of the weekend.

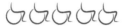

My friend James and his family were going to their house in Michigan for Memorial Day weekend, and I was invited. Only this time, my parents would not be going—Mr. Wilson had offered to help take care of me. My parents were a bit hesitant to agree, but after my insistence that everything would be fine, they relented. It would be the first time I ever went away overnight by myself.

After the grueling drive to Michigan, naturally, the first order of business was to head to the pool—the house had a very nice patio and pool area, with an in-ground pool. After James's dad helped me change into swimming trunks, James pushed me in my manual wheelchair out to the pool. I had spent several minutes deciding how I would get in the pool when Mr. Wilson got a big smile on his face and said, "Here, let me help you with that." He proceeded to push my wheelchair up to the edge of the pool and tilt it forward until I fell in. I was accustomed to being treated like I was made of glass, so I oddly appreciated the shenanigans.

Later that night, it was raining, so we all stayed inside. Mr. Wilson was moderating an intense game of hide-and-seek. He was also my designated assistant when hiding. The best idea the two of us had was for me to hide on the top shelf of the linen closet. I had to contort a little to fit, but Mr. Wilson was able to get me up on the shelf relatively comfortably. The finishing touch was placing a stack of towels in front of me. I was practically invisible and was the last to be found. James's cousin eventually gave up trying to look.

All the kids—James, James's brother and sister, and a few cousins—teamed up to look for me and still couldn't do it. I could hear the adults' muffled voices saying, "Warmer... Colder... So close." When the kids were sufficiently frustrated, Mr. Wilson went straight to the closet and scooped me out. There was a collective groan from the other kids and a great feeling of satisfaction for me.

The next day, the plan was to take the kids down to the creek behind the house. There was a rope swing— enough said. The only issue was how to transport me on the unpaved, uneven, dirt trail. My manual wheelchair was not built for going off road, so another solution needed to be found. After a good deal of time, James's aunt came around the corner of the house with an old, rusty wheelbarrow and facetiously added "Your chariot awaits." My immediate response was, "I can't sit in that!" Mr. Wilson covered the inside with a folded tarp, and just like that, I had no more complaints; I had a means of transportation, albeit a dirty one, with more spiders than I would like.

After a surprisingly smooth ride, we arrived. I sat upright and was able to see James swing out and drop into the water. I began freaking out about how I was supposed to do the same. I nervously watched the other kids take their turns until it was mine.

Unbeknownst to me, Mr. Wilson had made some kind of low-tech harness out of several lengths of bungee cord or something. Before I could get a good look at it, he grabbed me out of the wheelbarrow and sat in the harness. With me clutched in his arms, he jumped, and away we went.

We both landed in the water, and I untensed upon realizing I was okay. I was relieved to find this was the most exciting part of the weekend.

CHAPTER FIVE

AN INCONVENIENT TRUTH

PART ONE: HIGH SCHOOL BEGINS

My family received a lot of generous assistance from the community, allowing me to stay at my grade school. The principal stayed until I graduated, fellow students helped carry me up the stairs, and, not least of all, they built an elevator just for me. Could we realistically expect the same thing in high school?

We might have managed something similar if I went to the neighborhood high school—also a private, Catholic school—but there were no guarantees. I would instead be going to a public high school, where all the accommodations are required by law.

I had my choice to attend three or four different schools around the city, and I chose Jackson High School, which was considered the best at the time.

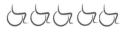

The only thing I remember about the first day of high school is waiting for my newly hired, one-on-one personal aide.[10]

---

10 My aide would be responsible for assisting me throughout the entire school day.

My parents and I sat in the special education director's office and waited. And waited. As if I wasn't nervous enough, I now had plenty of time to imagine what my new aide would be like. Considering my brief experience at Lincoln School, I didn't have high hopes.

When I did finally see my aide, I was slightly relieved. Frank was a young, Hispanic man in his mid-twenties; he was dressed casually, and had a very laid-back demeanor. This guy was definitely an improvement over the aides at Lincoln school.

As I was sizing up my new aide, my parents were summoned to another room to sign paperwork. The overly smiley woman who came to escort my parents, proclaimed in an unnecessarily enthusiastic tone of voice, "We'll leave you two alone to get to know each other!" We both smiled awkwardly, waiting for her to walk away.

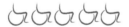

I was honestly not interested in getting to know Frank as a person; I was more concerned with the logistics of having an aide. I asked nervously, "How does this work?" He replied, "I don't know. I guess we'll have to figure that out." I wasn't satisfied with that answer and tried a more specific question, "Well, do you sit in class with me or just carry my books?" He answered similarly, "I don't know, do you want me to sit in class with you?"

After a few more questions, I began to realize I would

have a significant amount of control over how Frank helped me. That was exciting; it would be nice to have some autonomy. But, on the other hand, I was accustomed to having my parents take care of everything for me. It would be quite a big change.

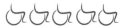

I wouldn't realize it until much later, but adjusting to high school was a lot more difficult for me than it was for my peers. In addition to the typical hurdles—getting acclimated to a new environment, using lockers, making friends, I was also faced with obstacles specific to having a disability.

For starters, I was simply trying to get comfortable asking Frank, more or less a complete stranger, for everything I needed. I also struggled to explain my preferences, such as how I liked to use the bathroom, or how I wanted my lunch set up.[11]

With all the extra issues to address, the social and academic sides of high school were inadvertently pushed to the background. When I am nervous about asking to use the bathroom too many times in a day, everything else seems less important.

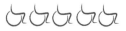

---

11 I needed my food prepared in a particular way to allow me to feed myself. This included: my sandwich cut in half, a straw in my drink, and everything close together so I could reach it.

For several weeks, it seemed like nothing was changing. The boundaries with Frank were unclear, and I was still learning the logistics of having an aide. It was extremely slow going, but eventually there was a breakthrough.

One day, as I waited for my computer class to start, Frank asked what video games I liked. I told him that I played *Madden* football. His response was a pleasant surprise: "Me too! I play online all the time. The Colts are my *team*." I wasn't sure how much of a gamer he was, so I tested the waters. "I don't know, the Colts don't have a good defense in that game, and Peyton Manning is too slow." He came back with, "I hear you. Sometimes I switch it up and play with the Falcons. Michael Vick is one of the fastest players in the game."

I was thrilled Frank and I had found something to bond over; and I would soon discover we had a lot more in common. We both liked sports, we both played fantasy football, we both liked video games of all types, and on and on.

Once we started to develop a rapport, everything fell into place. I ceased to be nervous to ask for things, and Frank began to learn my preferences.

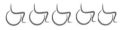

Now that I was relatively confident, I could meet my basic needs, my focus shifted toward making friends. Though, I wasn't entirely sure how to go about it. I was with the same group of kids from K–8; so, I was a bit rusty at making new friends, and understandably nervous.

Luckily, my first small victory was basically handed to me. Frank and I were sitting together at lunch, as we had since the school year began. All the while, I continued looking over at a particularly large group of freshmen: three or four tables pushed together, with about fifteen people sitting around them. In addition to being huge, it was also far more diverse than the other tables: goths, jocks, stoners, urban black kids, preppy white kids. All these freshmen had clearly congregated in solidarity. They hadn't yet separated into homogenous groups.

I sat there, only partially paying attention to my conversation with Frank, trying to work up the courage to go over there. As I debated with myself, a girl from the table came over and asked both of us if we would like to sit with them. I immediately said "YES," and was so excited I forgot to explain that Frank was not a student.

A few scattered, awkward verbal exchanges transpired, and it was clear no one was comfortable. I was relieved to see that my fellow freshmen were just as nervous as I was.

Knowing I wasn't alone gave me the confidence to put myself out there. The next day, I approached another freshman sitting by himself, in the cafeteria, and asked to join him. He said, "Sure," and just like that, I had a friend to eat lunch with. I started making an effort to talk to the girls I sat by in homeroom, and that seemed to go well. I even cracked a joke in my English class, and everyone laughed.

I was feeling pretty great, far from the terrifying uncertainty of the first day.

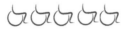

AN INCONVENIENT TRUTH

PART TWO: THE TRUTH HURTS

After the initial hurdles, I had fallen into a comfortably boring routine: I showed up in the morning; Frank carried my books to each class and helped me use the bathroom a few times; then, I returned home. It was the same thing every day, mundane but predictable.

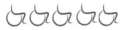

It was business as usual. I was suffering through yet another biology class, counting the minutes until lunch. As exciting as glycolysis is, I found myself bored and randomly flipping through the textbook as I waited for the bell.

I happened to come across a section in one of the later chapters that caught my attention. It was a section about Duchenne muscular dystrophy—my disability. I was genuinely curious, seeing as I didn't know anything about the actual biology behind it.

I read through the list of symptoms: muscle weakness— yes, falls for no apparent reason—yes, walks on the toes without the heels touching the ground—also completely accurate. It was pretty cool to see basically my entire experience with muscular dystrophy mapped out in textbook language.

I read a bit further: "The child with Duchenne has a characteristic way of rising from a seated or lying position. He places both feet apart and raises the torso so he is on all fours. The child then places his hands on his knees and pushes himself upright." I was surprised to learn that this was scientifically documented. I always thought that was simply the way I had found, through trial and error, to get up off the ground. It seemed every other kid with Duchenne had figured it out as well.

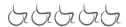

When I was near the end, I read the phrase "life-shortening" and instantly froze. I felt my heart beating through my ears, the teacher's voice shrinking to meaningless background noise. My mind was racing, barely processing the life-altering information. "That can't be true!"

Even though every word was excruciating, I needed to finish reading. I needed to know the truth, whatever it was.

As I continued, I saw the phrases "heart failure" and "respiratory failure." Then, I read the worst of it: "rarely survive beyond age eighteen." "Eighteen!?" Did I really only have three and a half years to live? This was news to me.

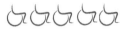

There I was, fourteen years old, sitting in class, having an existential crisis over my early mortality, desperately trying to hide what I was undergoing. Then, the bell rang. I still had four more hours of school. I wasn't sure how I was going to keep it together for the rest of the day.

The next period was lunch, and I don't think I said a word the entire time. There were swarms of thoughts, feelings, and questions flying through my head: "How could I not know this until now?" "Does my family know this?" "Do my parents assume I *already* know this?" "I guess it makes perfect sense. I never see any old people with Duchenne."

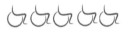

AN INCONVENIENT TRUTH

PART THREE: HARD TIMES

In a way, the experience of learning my prognosis mirrored the experience of my parents learning my diagnosis ten years earlier: the game of life came to a crashing halt, and all of my notions of the future were forever changed. The only difference was my parents were adults when they received their life-altering news; so, at the very least, they had some resilience. I was fourteen. I had nothing.

There was no chance for a healthy response, I had no means to process this. As the weeks went by, the only thing I could see was a hopeless situation. Any attempt to see things differently always ended with the same train of thought: "But then again, what is the point of X if I am only going to be dead in four years anyway?" "What is the point of anything?"

My emotional state slowly became darker and darker, as this hopelessness became my singular fixation. For the next several months, I sunk into a deep depression.

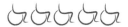

All that time, I never sought help. During my entire freshman year, I never talked to anyone. I believed no one could possibly understand what I was going through.

The way I understood seeking advice was to look to someone who has been through the same thing. Most kids my age had problems with girls, or needed pointers on how to throw a baseball, and had plenty of role models to look to; but, where were my role models? I didn't know anyone else with Duchenne.

I decided that going to someone was pointless. Instead, I chose to hide it. If I couldn't fix the problem, I would just ignore it. I would act like nothing was wrong and hope it went away.

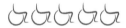

Eventually, all those negative feelings I was keeping bottled up would need to be let out.

Whenever my emotions reached the tipping point, which happened at least once a week, they would all come pouring out.

This took the form of crying myself to sleep. My mom would get me ready for bed, and I would do my best to keep it together until she was finished. Once the lights went off and she left the room, it would begin. I would start bawling and do my best to keep quiet so no one would hear.

As time went on, the downward spiral continued, and the severity of my symptoms magnified. I would start to develop physical symptoms that weren't as easy to hide.

It started suddenly one day, on my way to school. I felt a warm sensation in my stomach and had little time to react, as I quickly leaned over to throw up on the side of the school bus. The driver asked if I was sick, and I said rather perplexed, "I guess so. It must have been something I ate."

A few days later, it happened again in computer class. I was working on the day's assignment, as usual, when I felt that same, warm sensation again. "That can't be what it is. Not again." I ignored it and kept working. Then, without warning, I threw up all over my desk. The room fell silent; I didn't say a word and slowly made my way toward the door.

As I headed to the bathroom to clean up, that warm feeling started creeping up again and I knew it wasn't over yet. I frantically zoomed to the bathroom, and when I realized I wasn't going to make it, I leaned to the side and hoped for the best. Still barreling down the hall at full speed, I successfully left a long trail of puke behind me.

I kept thinking as long as I made it to the bathroom, I could still minimize the damage. But by the time I finally got to the bathroom, I was empty.

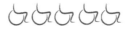

It soon became clear I wasn't simply sick to my stomach, as I began to throw up every day like clockwork. My mom tried to attribute it to this or that: eating before bed, what I ate for breakfast, or motion sickness from the school bus. But she never found the cause.

Of course, I knew exactly why this was happening; I just didn't want to admit it. Blaming my throwing up on eating pizza before bed was much easier than admitting I was depressed. And since we weren't addressing the real problem, on and on it went.

Getting sick became part of my daily school routine. I would arrive, and run to the bathroom; Frank would wait until I came back, and we would continue our day without drawing attention to it. There was always a possibility of a second occurrence, and this too was dealt with quietly.

It happened so often that we started to get desensitized. Even the occasional unexpected incident didn't faze either of us. One time I threw up in the hall, while heading to my next class, and never even slowed down. I heard some girl ask, "Oh my God, is he okay?" Frank waved her off and said nonchalantly, "He's fine." We both continued to the class unaffected.

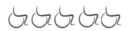

AN INCONVENIENT TRUTH

PART FOUR: MOVING FORWARD

After months of hiding my depression, crying, and throwing up all the time, I was burned out. I had absolutely no energy to deal with these problems, and thought about ending it all.

Even though it was a fleeting thought and I never had any intention to follow through, I was still scared. Was I in danger of harming myself? Could I trust myself to be left alone? Had my depression turned into full-blown mental illness? It felt like this new development was a harbinger of terrible things to come. But, little did I know, it was quite the opposite. This one fleeting thought would be the catalyst for bringing an end to my depression.

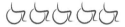

Over the previous several months, I had become numb to all the negativity. I was accustomed to passively accepting all of my dark and depressing thoughts, letting anything enter into my mind, and stay there as long as it wanted. But this time, it was different. I felt myself pushing back; part of me just could not allow such a dark thought to pass unchallenged.

I had rejected this one negative thought, and that was all it took to begin the chain reaction; over the next few days, I rejected another negative thought, and then another and another, until eventually there were no negative thoughts left. It was very strange, how quick the change happened.

The connection had been severed, and I could feel the depression gradually drifting farther and farther away, until it disappeared completely.

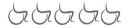

It was time to actually deal with my situation. I was finally ready to accept that my disability was life-shortening, and move on. The only problem was I didn't know what that looked like. Where did I begin? What was the first step?

After some contemplation, I decided to do some research

into Duchenne. I figured the best place to start was gathering information. If I was going to accept my situation, I needed to know exactly what I was dealing with.

It was immediately confirmed that my high school textbook had been correct—it was a life-shortening condition. However, I started to see cases of people living well past eighteen, into their late twenties and early thirties. I realized eighteen was actually the *average life expectancy*, not an absolute guarantee. I started to think, "My situation is above average: I have supportive parents, access to good healthcare, and excellent insurance. So, the average life expectancy won't necessarily apply to me."

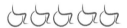

This new revelation was a pleasant surprise. It wasn't fantastic news, but it was enough to make me hopeful. For the first time in over a year, I was optimistic about the future.

CHAPTER SIX

COLLEGE?

The Muscular Dystrophy Association (MDA) hosts a week-long summer camp every year for all of its kids. It is a simple idea: give kids with MD the opportunity to have a typical summer camp experience that might otherwise be impossible.[12] I always looked forward to it all year, and was sad when it was over.

It was a constant party. We yelled chants in the cafeteria. Music played constantly. There was always something fun and exciting to do, be it wheelchair hockey or basketball, arts and crafts, a carnival night, a dance, or entertainment, such as a police dog demo or cosplay medieval battle.

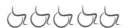

My favorite part of camp was the atmosphere. All the volunteers and counselors had the motto: "camp is for the campers," and it was evident in all aspects of the camp. We would play wheelchair hockey on the unshaded blacktop, and there would be an army of volunteers ready to give us

12 Each kid with MD is considered a "camper," and gets one volunteer "counselor," or one-on-one personal aide, for the week. Typical cabins and camp activities are also made accessible.

all water and sunscreen, as though we were professional athletes. If a group of us wanted to play a board game, someone would suddenly appear with a pile of options: Risk, Monopoly, Connect Four.

They even acknowledged the "little victories" that often go unnoticed. One night, I was sitting at the cafeteria table, waiting for dinner. The staff did not usually wait to serve the food, and I was getting impatient. I was starving after a day of wheelchair hockey in the summer heat: a level of hunger I wasn't familiar with, as I didn't usually physically exert myself. My mouth was watering at the thought of whatever crappy food they were serving for dinner this time, but still we waited.

Then, I started hearing a commotion outside. People were clapping and yelling like they had just encountered a famous person. I couldn't easily get up and run to the door, so I strained my neck trying to see.

After several minutes, nothing had happened. I was getting annoyed, and began asking some of the camp workers, "Why can't we have our food yet?" "Seriously, what is going on?" "Is it *that* important?" They were being dismissive and "shhh-ing" me like a small child in church, as if I was somehow being disrespectful.

The cheering gradually became louder and louder, with significantly more voices joining in. I heard someone shout, "Awesome job!" I heard another voice shout, "Here he comes! You are almost there!" I heard the final cathartic roar of the crowd, and then a kid dragged his way into the cafeteria with his walker.

After the cheers died down, one of the camp administrators got on the microphone, reserved for nightly announcements, and exclaimed, "Aaron walked all the way from his cabin to the cafeteria! That is half a mile! Let's give him a round of applause!" The whole cafeteria cheered even louder than before.

I suddenly felt guilty for being so impatient. Walking a half-mile for someone of this kid's ability, was quite a physical feat. It was great to see something that would usually only be appreciated by a parent, being praised by the entire camp.

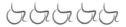

Every year, I couldn't wait to go to camp. When the end of each school year approached, I began counting down the days. But, this year, I wasn't as thrilled. It had been a difficult several months, struggling with depression and trying to process what I had learned about my disability. I felt drained, and was generally not up for a big social event.

I told my parents I didn't want to go, and they looked puzzled. My mom said with concern in her voice, "But you love going to camp. Why don't you want to go?" I quickly realized "I don't feel like it" wasn't a good enough answer, and after several weeks of pestering, I reluctantly agreed to return to camp.

This turned out to be one of the best decisions I ever made. A guest speaker visited camp that year. Her name was Lauren Kincaid, and she had quite an amazing story to tell. Lauren also had MD, and had just recently graduated from Generic Midwest University (not the real name). The part that was thrilling to me was she was able to live on campus, away from home. She had apparently stayed at an adaptive dorm, which allowed people of her, and my, level of disability to easily live independently. That was when I learned about Roberts, the specialized residential program at Generic Midwest University.

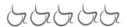

I had never given college much thought up until then, assuming it would just be four more years of the same school experience: getting up early, catching a ride, going to class, and coming back home. It was always a given that "away-from-home college" was not in the cards for me. But when I heard Lauren Kincaid talk about Roberts, I could suddenly see that as a real possibility.

I returned home and told my parents I wanted to go away to school as nonchalantly as asking the time. My dad likes to remind me of "…the time you came home from camp and told me you wanted to go away to college, we thought it sounded like a nice idea, but it was impossible."

To them, my decision was made in a manner similar to when a small child talks about their future career.

When a little kid says they want to be an astronaut when they grow up, they don't comprehend what it takes to get there. They haven't the faintest clue of how much education, hard work, or sacrifice it takes to achieve their goal. In the same way, my parents assumed I decided to go away to school without really understanding what it takes to get there.

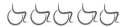

As "ridiculous" as it sounded: the idea of someone with my level of disability going away to school, I think my parents were still intrigued by the idea. After researching the Roberts program out of sheer curiosity, it seemed legitimate. But still, it sounded too good to be true. People of my level of disability could not live on their own, could they? There had to be a catch.

At each step in the process, they were both just waiting to find the part where it wouldn't work out. Would the rooms be accessible? Would there be anyone available to help me in the middle of the night? How would I hit the elevator button to get to my classes? Something had to be wrong.

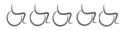

We never encountered that deal-breaker on the website. It

was time to drive down to GMU and see what this Roberts program was all about. So, one July afternoon, we took a road trip down there.

We met with Sharon, the Roberts administrator, and my mom had a lot of questions for her. "Who will take care of him?" "The program provides personal assistants (PAs) for all personal care needs." "Where do you get the PAs?" "They are students also." My mom's fear was growing. "How are PAs assigned to residents?" "The resident is entirely responsible for scheduling their own PAs." My mom's fear was still rising. "Well, how will I know he will be okay?" "You will just have to trust him." Now her fear had turned into complete and utter terror.

My mom was nearly in tears expressing all her concerns about her baby. And Sharon didn't even flinch. She had a good answer for every question, and delivered each answer like she had done it hundreds of times before. Terrified parents were likely a regular occurrence at these meetings.

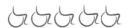

After speaking with the Roberts administrator, we went to the disability services office and met with each department head: testing accommodations, physical therapy, transportation, academic accommodations, and on and on. In terms of the services they offered, each office we visited was more impressive than the last.

With each successive meeting, going away to school became more and more realistic; the look of curious disbelief in my mother's face, was replaced by a look of palpable fear. She had realized I very well could move out of the house and go away to school.

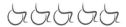

Our last stop was the financial aid office. We met with Jim, the case manager for something called the Federal Ticket to Work Program. This basically meant he was the one in charge of ensuring the government paid for my tuition. He was the most important person we visited that day.

Jim was more than just another bureaucrat; he had a wisdom about him. He was like the Yoda or Gandalf of the disability services office, a wise old sage who had been around longer than anyone.

He had started working there in the late 1950s, and had a lot of stories to share. Jim told us how disability services at Generic Midwest University began as part of the G.I. Bill, a way to help wounded World War II veterans go to college. He told us how the wheelchair basketball team was started to help vets get exercise. Jim continued to tell us about all the ground-breaking innovations Generic Midwest University had initiated. Curb cuts were invented to allow wheelchair-using students to cross the street easily. GMU was also the first place, anywhere in the world, to have a mechanical wheelchair lift on a bus—a mechanical engineering student helped design it—and consequently, the first place to have wheelchair-accessible bus routes.

Jim's biggest insight was about the Roberts program itself. I'll never forget what he said: "A lot of people think it is discrimination, putting all the disabled students in one place. But, it's not. They learn from each other and relate to each other in a way they couldn't with able-bodied students."

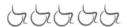

The three of us left astonished. We were shown something that had previously seemed impossible. Even I, who was the most optimistic, couldn't believe it. The idea of going to college sounded nice on paper, but I didn't fully believe it until I saw it for myself.

After learning I could actually go away to college, I was reinvigorated with new purpose. I didn't just want to get into GMU, I needed to.

CHAPTER SEVEN

NEW BEGINNINGS

PART ONE: ANTICIPATION

I was extremely thorough in preparing for the GMU application. I retook the ACT twice, and worked on my essay, for weeks, to ensure it would be perfect. And, everything on my application was spotless, except for one thing: the extracurriculars.

Dealing with depression, I had not made an effort to engage in extracurricular activities; and now it was coming back to haunt me. Even if I wanted to join some things, it was already too late. Applications were due by December, and it was now the beginning of November. I had to just submit it as it was.

I fluffed up my resume the best I could, and submitted what I had, hoping the admissions board would find a way to take pity on me.

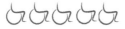

The uncertainty was agonizing. I probably checked the online application, every two hours, for several weeks.

After an excruciating month of constant checking and waiting, I loaded up my online application and saw the following words: "decision made: yes." I held my breath, knowing as soon as I drifted my eyes a few millimeters to the right, I would know. Then I saw it. I saw the word "accepted."

Getting into GMU was exactly what I wanted, but my reaction was not typical. I wasn't thrilled, nor did I run to tell my parents the good news. Instead, I sat silently at my computer, relieved that I had not ruined this amazing opportunity.

Then, when my existential relief died down, I finally started to feel the usual excitement and elation. I told my parents, but their reaction was not typical either; they were not so much excited as they were terrified.

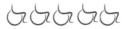

Before I even had time to let the news sink in, my parents started worrying. They began sharing their concerns on a daily basis. I endured the next few months of "Are you sure you want to go there?" "They won't take care of you as good as I can." It got to the point where I wasn't sure which feeling was stronger: my own anxieties about college or my frustration with my parents' anxieties.

I could not understand why they were so afraid. They kept telling me I wasn't taking it seriously enough, but, in my mind, I absolutely was. I had concerns too: scheduling

PAs, [13] making friends, finding my way around campus; I was just not losing my mind with fear like they were.

I didn't think there was any reason to start worrying about moving in until at least late July. A few weeks was all I would need to get everything in order.

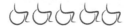

I thought I had everything under control, but I would soon get a literal wake-up call that I did not. One day, the Roberts administrator called my house. My mom answered, and I got an earful after she hung up. "Sharon said she has been sending important emails to all the incoming residents, and you're the only one who hasn't been responding!" "You have to start contacting PAs! They are the only reason you're able to go away to school!"

With the combination of the admin actually calling my house, and my mom setting me straight, I began to take preparing for school more seriously. I promptly started contacting prospective PAs, talking to current Roberts residents, and connecting with my future suitemate.[14]

As I began to hear of managing PAs, figuring out how to allot my five PA hours per day, and scheduling them around my classes, it was clear I had not realized what an undertaking this college thing was going to be. I thought,

---

13 Recall that a PA, short for personal assistant, helps with personal care needs. PAs would be my primary caregivers at school.

14 The Roberts rooms were split into pairs, with one shared bathroom.

"I have to do all of that, and then make time for homework and fun things?"

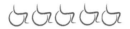

NEW BEGINNINGS

PART TWO: ARRIVAL

At long last, the day had arrived. We packed up the van and hit the road. There was officially no turning back now.

We arrived on campus, and pulled up to Roberts Hall. The unimpressive, sixty-year-old building, with its red-brick façade and rickety wooden balconies, was going to be my new home.

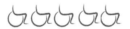

As I was using the wheelchair lift to disembark, we were greeted by Sharon. She directed me inside, and the whirlwind started before my parents were even inside. I arrived at a desk with several orientation forms to fill out. Then, I had to take an ID picture and sign a liability waiver. Next, I signed a room condition report and spoke to the student mentors. It was dizzying, but the real stress was yet to come: my parents still needed to get my new room together.

As my dad began carrying things in, I listened to all of

my mom's concerns while she was frantically unpacking. "Do you have your room key?" "Can we rearrange the furniture?" "Where do you think is the best place to put your towels?" "I can't believe I'm leaving my baby here by himself!" I was overwhelmed to say the least.

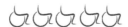

Though it seemed to go on forever, the initial rush had finally passed, and it was now time for the new student/ parent welcome meeting. The other nine new students and I waited apprehensively, with our parents, for Sharon to begin. This was the first time I saw all my new dormmates in the same place. I took the opportunity to size them up.

The only place similar to Roberts I had experienced was MDA camp, so all my expectations stemmed from that. I had half-expected all of the people at Roberts to look like campers at MDA camp, but quickly realized the error of that assumption.

The guy, sitting across from me, was essentially lying down in his wheelchair. The guy to my right, decked out in Miami sports attire, was actively using his arms, though his fingers seemed to be stuck in place. I saw a guy, who obviously didn't have any muscle weakness, push himself through the door in a manual wheelchair, followed by his service dog.

In the middle of eyeing my new classmates, Sharon entered and instructed us to introduce ourselves. One girl introduced herself as a graduate student, and the guy next to her as her fiancée. "Did she just say fian—" My thought was interrupted by the next girl saying she was a transfer student from Boston College. She had been paralyzed in a car accident and transferred to GMU for the Roberts program. "Wow that is nuts! I wonder what—" My thought was interrupted again by the next girl. I couldn't really understand what she was saying. It seemed her voice was a bit distorted by her disability and, by the look on her face, talking seemed strenuous for her. I was tempted to assume she was kind of slow, but then I remembered she was a college student just like me. "I wonder how often people assume she is slow—" My thought was interrupted by Sharon moving on to the next part of the meeting.

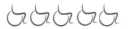

I was starting to get bored of the welcome-to-college routine, but then Sharon started saying some things that resonated with me: "You have all gotten this far. You have gotten into this program, but your job is not done yet. If you do nothing but go to and from class, you will be wasting your money." She had a message for the parents as well: "If you feel you have adequately prepared your son or daughter to succeed in life, then you have nothing to worry about. It is time to let them make their own decisions; some of them may even come home with tattoos and earrings. I remember one girl; she would often eat chocolate cake for breakfast. Whatever it is, the time has come to let them learn for themselves."[15] At this, several mothers gasped.

The rest of the meeting was uneventful, filled with rules and logistics. I was just happy when it was over. I had been going all day, and the pizza that was served for dinner seemed heavenly.

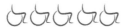

The emotional tsunami of my first day was coming to a close, but all the "firsts" were still not over. This would be my first night, away at school, without my parents.

Though it had been explained in the welcome meeting, I was completely blanking on how the night system worked. I asked the PA putting me to bed, who explained that repositioning people at night was the floater's job. I learned that the floater was the on-call PA available to all the residents through a wireless paging system. Different people clocked in and out every few hours, but there was always a floater on duty.

I ended up paging the night floater a few times, and it was a new experience trying to explain to a complete stranger how I like to reposition.

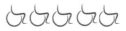

---

15 Many young people with disabilities are extremely sheltered. The idea that their child can be independent is unimaginable for some parents.

My parents were too concerned to just leave after the first night, so they stayed at a hotel and returned the next morning. They came back to show my PA how to do my routine; but it was done in such a panic, she did not really learn anything. "It was so early, and they were throwing so much information at me," she would later confess, "I didn't really catch any of it."

After this incredibly frantic and stressful morning, it was time for them to leave. I was excited to finally be on my own, but I will admit I was equally nervous. I followed my parents out to the van, and waited until they got in. After an emotional, tear-filled goodbye from my mother, I watched them drive away.

Suddenly, it hit me like a speeding semi: I was truly on my own. I returned to the cafeteria to finish my lunch, and didn't really know what to do next. I had done all of this work to prepare tor college, and now that I was here, what was I supposed to do?

I didn't have much time to ruminate on that, however, because I had an entire day filled with orientation meetings.

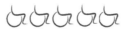

I had woken up at seven. I had just gone through the quasi-traumatic experience of my parents leaving. It was my first day, on my own, away from home, in a new place, and I didn't know anyone. I wasn't exactly in the best state of mind to pay attention during a bunch of meetings.

There were meetings one after the other, after the other, for eight hours. After the first two meetings, I had exhausted my quota of attention span for the day. But there were still transportation people, accommodation letter[16] people, campus police, campus fire department, and on and on. Each speaker was spitting out all these rules and protocols we were expected to remember, but I was tuned out.

The director of the disability services office imparted one of the few pieces of advice that actually stuck with me. She told us to be selfish with our PAs. This brought me out of my daydream. Selfish? What was she talking about?

It turns out, "being selfish" meant being assertive and speaking up for yourself. PAs were, after all, there to help us. We were technically their employers,[17] and had every right to have our needs met in a manner we saw fit. She said not to feel bad if we have to fire someone, not to feel afraid to ask our PAs for absolutely everything we need. She said bluntly, "PAs are here for you, and it's your job to tell them what you need. If you're shy or whatever, you need to get over it."

This was good advice, and I intended to follow it as best I could. However, I would soon regret not paying attention to the rest of the advice I had been given that day.

---

16 Each student was to have a letter describing which academic accommodations they needed. They would then give the letter to their professors.

17 Recall that residents are solely in charge of scheduling their PAs. They are also responsible for screening, hiring, and managing their PAs.

CHAPTER EIGHT

A STEEP LEARNING CURVE

The instant my parents left, any sense of normalcy and equilibrium left with them. All of a sudden, I was on my own, learning to manage my own life. I had no idea what I was doing. And, for the first few months, I was plagued with a constant feeling of uneasiness.

ᎧᎧᎧᎧᎧ

A STEEP LEARNING CURVE

PART ONE: TRIAL AND ERROR

The biggest hurdle was learning to manage my PAs. At Roberts, I was expected to evaluate potential caregivers, decide who to hire, and, not least of all, teach them how to help me.

In the past, the majority of my personal care had been handled by my mother, and I never had to teach her anything. I suddenly found people looking to me for direction. I had no idea how to explain the best way to lift me, or position me in my wheelchair.

ᓇᓇᓇᓇᓇ

PA shifts took a long time to get through at first. Finding a good explanation for each task was a slow process. They would ask, "What's the best way to clip your fingernails?" And it was like rocket science: trying to find the perfect formula, the magic words my PA would understand.

It always took several attempts to explain anything. If I tried to tell someone how to put my shirt on, for example, I would begin with simple directions: "move my arm toward you" or, "pull my hand out of the sleeve." When the initial explanations failed, I would then have to test different phrases and word choices. If "pull my hand out of the sleeve" didn't work, then maybe "pull my arm out of the sleeve" was better, or "grab by the hand and pull away from my body."

I would often get frustrated because I could easily visualize what I wanted them to do, I just couldn't articulate it. But with persistence, I would always find the heart of the issue. With the shirt, it was my elbows. My elbows can not straighten all the way, and I realized that my PAs would try to force them straight to get my arm through the sleeve. Once I figured this out, my instruction became: "pull my arm out of the sleeve, but don't try to straighten the elbow;" and, just like that, the problem was solved.

It was always satisfying to find the right words, but I never had time to enjoy each little victory. As soon as I finished one task, it was on to the next.

Through trial and error, I started to refine my PA vocabulary. Instructing people was becoming easier, and shifts were getting shorter. But, in addition to logistics, it was also a matter of just being comfortable with the person. I now had complete strangers helping me use the bathroom, shower, and get dressed. Being assisted with such intimate tasks requires a lot of trust, and I was slow to warm up.

To make matters worse, my PAs were college students. The fact my caregivers were people my own age made the whole situation doubly awkward. I had a particular mental schema about what a caregiver was supposed to be: old, maybe a family member or a nurse—someone with a warm, comforting presence. They certainly weren't my peers.

Then, to make matters even worse than that, most of my PAs were girls. It was expected that residents would be mature enough to handle being taken care of by someone of the opposite sex, but I definitely wasn't. I was an eighteen-year-old guy who, up until that point, had never even kissed a girl before; they were still scary, unknown creatures. And, all of a sudden, I was supposed to get naked in front of them?! I didn't want some pretty girl seeing everything.

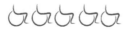

For the first week, I had been avoiding being showered by any girls. I went out of my way to only shower with male PAs, doing ridiculous things like: waiting several days until my next male PA, and showering in the middle of the day. But, by Friday morning, I couldn't avoid it any longer. It was really hot outside and I absolutely needed to shower, regardless of who my PA was.

Friday morning rolled around, and I woke up to the faint sound of footsteps outside my room. The door creaked open, and I heard someone enter. I slowly opened my eyes and couldn't believe what I saw: this goddess digging through my dresser drawer. Not only was she stunning; she was also dressed for the season: short shorts and a low-cut tank top. For a moment, I was so captivated I couldn't think straight. Then she turned to talk to me, and I immediately started to panic.

I was so embarrassed I completely avoided eye contact, and mumbled all my instructions. My voice shook as I told her I needed to shower. She asked, "Should I take your underwear off now?" The panic intensified. "Oh no, that sounds like dialogue from a low-quality porno movie!!" I was telling myself over and over: "Don't think bad thoughts." "Don't think bad thoughts." And I managed to keep it together, as I got undressed and into the shower.

Things were going surprisingly well, but when it came time to wash "down there," I knew it was just a matter of time. All I could do was take a deep breath, and brace myself for the humiliation to come.

Then, to my relief and astonishment, nothing happened. In fact, there was not one awkward occurrence during the entire shift. Everything, from start to finish, was strangely innocuous.

Immediately after this incident, my attitude changed. It became abundantly clear that caregiving was entirely asexual; it was a practical task with the sole purpose of meeting my basic needs. The only thing that could make it weird was me.

ᕕᕕᕕᕕᕕ

A STEEP LEARNING CURVE

PART TWO: GROWING PAINS

As mentioned before, my parents had been my primary caregivers all my life. I was accustomed to interacting with them. They understood my directions, and knew my preferences. We had developed a comfortable routine. So naturally, when I moved to Roberts, I tried to replicate it. Most of the elements of my home routine transferred smoothly, but I had also carried over some bad habits

With my parents, there had been a lot of leniency with the way I asked for help. I never needed to consider if I was annoying or rude because my parents always ended up doing it. So, there was no incentive to start saying "please" and "thank you," and I never bothered to phrase my requests in the form of a question. Blunt, forceful directions like: "That isn't right," and "No, not like that," may have worked just fine at home, but they were not taken very kindly at Roberts.

My behavior was taken as rude, and people assumed I was a jerk. But, with all of these bad habits, I was never purposely disrespecting anyone. I had only ever known one way of interacting with my caregivers. Regardless of the reason, the fact remained: I was not treating my PAs with enough respect.

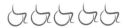

The negative reception to my behavior was swift and harsh. Several floaters called me out for not asking nicely. Another girl reprimanded me for jokingly implying she was doing a bad job. Yet another time, I overheard one of my PAs complaining about me through the wall.

The message was clear: I could not talk to my PAs the same way I talked to my parents. I immediately started changing my ways: phrasing requests for help as questions, as well as saying "please" and "thank you." And, lo and behold, I started getting better reactions from people. The complaints all but completely stopped.

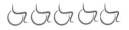

At the time, I thought people had been unreasonable, but,

in hindsight, this experience was good for me. My disability was no longer an excuse for unacceptable behavior. In the past, any unusual or awkward behavior could have been overlooked, pardoned because I was in a wheelchair and "couldn't help it." But here, everyone had a disability; PAs and residents alike weren't afraid to call someone out when they weren't acting right.

It might have seemed harsh, but if I had not been confronted, I wouldn't have been forced to grow and change. That kind of social reinforcement was exactly what I needed.

CHAPTER NINE

PROGRESS

PART ONE: MY NEW ROUTINE

I don't wake up to an alarm. The PA who comes to wake me up is the first thing I hear. She gets me dressed, lifts me into my wheelchair, brushes my teeth, and combs my hair. There is minimal conversation because we are both tired.

After forty-five minutes of the morning drudgery, I am hungry. Before leaving, she pours my cereal and sets up my breakfast. I have ten minutes to scarf down a bowl of Cheerios and get ready for the bus. Fortunately, the bus picks up right outside of Roberts, so I don't have far to go.

As I approach the main entrance, I can see, through the window, that the weather looks nice. I decide to forgo the bus and "walk" to class. I ride in the street because the sidewalks are filled with treacherous potholes and bumps.

I get to Nelson Hall and mentally prepare myself for calculus class. Nelson is the oldest building on campus; it's regarded as one of the landmarks of the University, but every time I am there it still seems like a dump. I flag down a random good Samaritan classmate to hit the elevator button for me.

It is difficult to stay awake in class at ten in the morning, but I fight the urge to sleep because the accessible seating is in the front row; I don't want the teacher to catch me sleeping in the middle of her riveting proof of Euler's Law. The bell rings. I flag down someone to get the elevator again, and return to Roberts for lunch.

I fly through the automatic doors, wheelchair at full speed, and make a beeline for the cafeteria. I've learned to get back and order my lunch,[18] as soon as possible, to minimize the wait. With the time I save, I can squeeze a PA shift in[19] while my usual chicken is on the grill.

As soon as I order my lunch, I go back to the Roberts lobby to fetch my PA. I quickly use the bathroom and return to lunch, just in time to find my food waiting for me. One of the meal assistants[20] had already brought my tray back to the table, and cut the sandwich in half. It really is the little things that get you through the day!

After lunch, it is time to head back out to my next class. I arrive early to Burton Hall, and wait outside the doors for the bell to ring. Even though it is a rhetoric class, the teacher makes it interesting. Regardless, I still get bored and start watching the clock. I have twenty minutes until I am free of all responsibility for the day.

I get back from class, and look for people to order

---

18 Due to its small size—about 30 residents—Roberts relied on one short-order cook for all meals.

19 Bathroom breaks needed to be strategically scheduled, so I didn't go all day without going to the bathroom.

20 The meal assistants are PAs that work during meal times, to help residents get set up with their food.

dinner with. Roberts is a small program, and isn't part of University Housing, so the food budget is tiny; hence, dinners are crap. I had quickly learned to avoid the dull, gray, vegetable medley, and "Salisbury steak." Instead, I ordered takeout just about every night.

I find Phil and Ron in the computer lab and suggest pizza. They agree. I hang out with Phil and Ron until our food arrives. My phone rings, but it falls on the floor as I try to answer it. We mildly panic, as none of us can reach the phone. Ron says jokingly, "Gravity... a cripple's worst enemy!"

I run to the floater desk,[21] and tell her I need my phone right away. She knows it is not as urgent as I make it seem and laughs, then comes with me to pick up the phone. The floater holds the phone up to my ear, so I can talk: it is the delivery guy.

As usual, they don't know where the main entrance is—Roberts is a small, nondescript building, and doesn't particularly look like a dorm. Ron volunteers to go outside and get him. You can see the awkwardness in his face: encountering a large group of wheelchairs intimidates most who are unfamiliar. I ask the floater to assist in giving him the money; then she brings the food into the cafeteria, where the meal assistants are waiting.

Dinners at Roberts are a time for everyone to unwind

---

21 Recall that the floater is available 24/7—not just at night—for small, incidental tasks. They are stationed at a desk, in the main lobby, so residents can easily find them.

after a busy day of class. The dining hall is the perfect place to hang out and relax: cozy, comfortable, more of a communal hub than a formal cafeteria. As usual, I hang out long after I finish eating. The after-dinner fraternizing is only interrupted by my PA showing up for his usual shower shift.

After my shower, I do homework, for an hour or two, until my night PA arrives. She gets me ready for bed—brushes my teeth, stretches my legs—but I remain dressed and in my wheelchair. One of the best things about living on my own is I have no set bedtime. The floater is always there and can throw me in bed whenever—a little trick of the trade I picked up.

I mingle with the other night owls until about two in the morning, and retire to bed safe in my assumption that tomorrow will follow a similar formula.

ⱴⱴⱴⱴⱴ

PROGRESS

PART TWO: GROWING CONFIDENCE

Once I mastered my day-to-day routine, my confidence was sky-high. I felt empowered to get out and see what else I was capable of.

ᴗᴗᴗᴗᴗᴗ

One night, Phil and I went to see the movie *Quantum of Solace*—all by ourselves. Neither of us had ever navigated public transportation on our own, but we were determined to figure it out. The two of us studied the bus routes as thoroughly as a sea captain about to embark on a trans-atlantic voyage; and after plotting the course, we headed out.

Phil and I arrived early and decided to eat at the Apple-bee's nearby. This was another first: eating at a restaurant on our own. Everything went smoothly, except for when I had to ask the waitress to reach in my pocket to get my wallet—that was a little awkward.

We went to buy the tickets, but neither of us could reach the counter. The cashier had to exit his little cubicle to help us complete the transaction, but he didn't seem to mind. Phil and I then waited outside of our theater for a fellow patron to open the door. After getting in and getting settled, we simply enjoyed the movie.

This was the first of many attempts to test the limits of my new independence. I found when it didn't require direct physical ability, there wasn't much I couldn't do. The logistics were always a bit improvised, and I often had to rely on the kindness of strangers or service sector employees, but I never let the obstacles stop me.

ᎶᎶᎶᎶᎶ

I was living it up, having all sorts of new experiences; I was enjoying all the aspects of going away to college. Well, all of the aspects except for one. But with the way I was jumping at every opportunity to do something new, it was only a matter of time before the inevitable happened.

A large group of us, including some off-duty PAs, went to the first football game of the season. The weather was still nice, and it was a perfect way to spend such a beautiful Saturday afternoon.

After the game, our guests wanted to go to Old Town for lunch. I had a PA shift, but planned to meet them after. An hour or so later, I made my way to Old Town only to discover it was a bar: Old Town Brewery.

I wasn't of-age and wondered, "Will they even let me in here?" I didn't know, I had never been to a bar. Luckily, I didn't have to find out: no one was at the door and I cruised right in.

Tom, the only able-bodied person there, offered me a beer from their pitcher. I had never drunk a drop of alcohol, and timidly refused. Alan and Ron immediately began pressuring me, but Tom quieted them down.

Then, *he* began pressuring me in a more sensitive manner: "You've never drank before?" I said, "No." "What's the reason?" I replied, "I don't know." "Yeah, you do, you must have a reason. Are you afraid? Or are you genuinely not interested?" Again, I timidly replied, "Well no, not exactly. I just didn't want to get in trouble." "I gotcha, your parents were always around, helping you and everything." I nodded. Tom replied, "Well you don't have to worry about that now, your parents aren't here." "I know, but I really shouldn't." "What's the worst that can happen?" I thought about it for a second, and he was absolutely right. My lack of parental supervision was a new luxury I needed to indulge.

I took a sip and paused. I thought to myself, "So that's what a beer tastes like." I took another drink: it was bitter and left a terrible aftertaste. I immediately told Tom I wanted no more. He replied in that same sensitive manner, "At least now you can say you tried it."

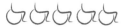

Honestly, I could have probably forced down a bit more, but I was also nervous. For one thing, I knew absolutely nothing about alcohol or drinking. All I could think of were scenes from those '90s high school movies: *She's All That, The 10 Things I Hate About You*, etc. In every party scene, there was always someone throwing up in the bathroom. I didn't want to be that person.

Furthermore, I had no idea what my limits were. It was clear Alan and Ron knew a little something about theirs; but I was still wondering, "Can I even drink? Will my body tolerate alcohol?" I didn't know if people with Duchenne can drink safely, and I wanted to be careful. I resolved to find my limits slowly and systematically.

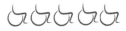

PROGRESS

PART THREE: COMMUNITY

As with high school previously, I focused more on getting the basics down before actively seeking out friends. For the first few weeks, all of my attention went to figuring out how to instruct my PAs and getting acclimated to the new environment. But now that I had reached those early milestones, I could relax and make more time for socializing.

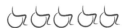

I got along well with several fellow freshmen, and a friend group formed seemingly overnight. I met my friend Ron, who liked anime as much as I did, and had an even stronger passion for video games. His eccentric tastes, quick wit, and grandiose ideas were a breath of fresh air. My suitemate Phil and I had the same disability, and immediately bonded over it. Then, of course, there was Alan, who was the Robin to my Batman.

The four of us just clicked. We were always together,

whether it was: during downtime, at meals, or out on the town. This was especially true on weekends. We were too young to drink and easily get away with it, so we didn't party a whole lot. But I don't think any of us really cared. We hung out every weekend and did our own thing: goofing off, watching movies, and playing hours and hours of *Super Smash Brothers*.

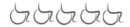

All of our bonding and time spent together formed the foundation for a strong sense of camaraderie. If one of us was having difficulty in a class, someone would offer help. If one of us wanted to share our opinion of something the administrator did, or of a floater we didn't like, it felt safe to share that. I eventually came to trust them like family. I knew I could go to them with any problem or issue and not be judged.

It was an enviable situation and I was grateful, especially because I never expected to have such a close friend group. In high school, making friends had been difficult for me, and I had hoped I could scrape together a few friends at Roberts. I never imagined I would make friends like these.

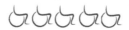

Through my new friend group, and just living at Roberts

in general, I found something I didn't know I was missing. For the first time, I felt that I could truly relate to my peers. Before Roberts, I had felt completely alone in my struggles, but now I was around people who understood exactly what I was going through.

I can still vividly remember the first time I realized I wasn't alone anymore. I had taken a stroll around town, with Ron, in an unsuccessful attempt to find a movie theater. On the way home, I casually asked him, "How are you adjusting?" and this basically opened the floodgates. I think, in a way, we had both been waiting for this conversation long before we ever came to Roberts.

Ron was quick to answer, "I'm doing okay. I know it's only been a week, but it's already better than high school." Ron explained, "I had a really hard time for a while. I was so angry all the time. I was constantly mad at everything I couldn't do. And, I lost a lot of friends." I couldn't believe his experiences were so similar to mine: "Oh my God! I know exactly what you mean. I was really quiet and shy in high school. And, I didn't really make any friends. But I think you're right, it is going to be better. It's going to be different now. It's all new, and we can reinvent ourselves here."

Ron continued, "Yeah that's true, it's an opportunity to start over. But I have to be careful not to fall into old habits. I could easily stay in my room all the time and play video games. And, I could be content doing that, but I don't want to be." I replied gratefully, "Me either. Wow! It's nice to know it's not just me!"

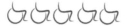

It was incredibly therapeutic to learn that my new friends had experienced similar difficulties. Though, as time went on, I found far more examples of experiences different from my own. Some people faced challenges and difficulties I never even knew existed. And the more I learned about my fellow Roberts residents, the more perspective I gained on my own situation.

The first thing that stuck out to me was a conversation I had with a resident about his cerebral palsy, or CP for short. He had casually mentioned that he was going to take a bus to a building two blocks away. I asked why, and explained he could just go two blocks east. He replied, "I would get lost. I'm terrible with directions. People with CP usually are." "What do you mean?" I asked. "It's poor spatial skills. Most people with CP are bad with directions and anything else that requires spatial reasoning, like math."

Additionally, I found that most of the Roberts residents had been in a wheelchair since birth. That alone was crazy to me. But it was only the beginning, the list went on: some of my new dormmates had trouble speaking, others had no sensation in their lower body. Some of them couldn't move their fingers, and some of them had to be on a strict bathroom routine.

Even Phil, who shared the same disability, had to deal with issues that I never did. We had an interesting conversation not too long after we met.

Phil and I had volunteered at the library, as part of the freshman seminar class, and spent several hours together. We were checking that the correct DVDs were in the correct boxes—conversation was the only way to escape the soul-crushing boredom. It started with some "getting-to-know-you" small talk, but after an hour or two we got into more heavy stuff.

I asked Phil, "Did you do the spinal fusion?"[22] Phil answered matter-of-factly, "Yea. You didn't?" I was somewhat uncomfortable answering: "No my heart function isn't good enough to withstand the procedure." He reassured me, "It's ok. It sucked honestly. I was in the hospital for weeks. The recovery was terrible, I had to have morphine constantly." He paused briefly, and continued: "Now I have to use a lift;[23] I can't easily be picked up and carried like you. And my spine has so many pins and screws in it, my x-ray looks like the frickin' Eifel Tower!" I added facetiously, "Oh yeah, well mine looks like a squiggly letter 'S!'[24] So, I win."

---

22 The spinal fusion is a surgery to correct scoliosis. It is a huge ordeal, involving attaching metal screws to the spine.

23 A Hoyer lift is a simple, hydraulic device that assists caregivers with lifting.

24 I had and still have severe spinal lordosis.

I started to feel grateful for some of the things I didn't have to deal with. I was glad I could find my way around without getting lost, I was glad I could use my fingers, and I was glad I didn't have to use a mechanical lift. The idea that my situation was by no means the absolute worst-case scenario was comforting in a way. Being fortunate was never something I had associated with having my disability.

CHAPTER TEN

CULTURE SHOCK

Roberts was its own little isolated subculture. It had its own rules, customs, and an entirely unique vocabulary. And at the very heart of it all was an extremely disability-positive attitude, unlike anything I had encountered before.

From day one, I was seduced. I couldn't get enough of this Roberts culture. I was like a sponge: soaking up as much of it as I could.

ひひひひひ

CULTURE SHOCK

PART ONE: LEARNING A SECOND LANGUAGE

The new terminology was the first thing I picked up on. I heard a plethora of new words, alternate definitions of words, and even some brand-new concepts. These ranged from describing everyday occurrences, to broad social implications for people with disabilities. For instance, "pee math" refers to the difficulty of trying to schedule all of your bathroom breaks throughout the day: if I were to drink X amount of liquid, then I could wait Y amount of time before having to go again. Then there was "inspiration porn." This refers to the media's bias for portraying people with disabilities as inspirational. This portrayal is considered exploitation in the same way pornography exploits young girls.

The terms used to describe each other were more endearing. Instead of the dry, politically-correct "wheelchair-user," the term "wheelie" was used. Paraplegics were "paras," while quadriplegics were "quads." Even able-bodied people were sometimes called "walkies."

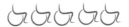

Of all the concepts I learned from this new dialect, my personal favorite was the "Crip Card." Before I explain what it is, I think I should give some background on this one.

People with disabilities are often treated with kid gloves. This was well understood by everyone: new students and seasoned veterans alike. It was also well understood that this behavior wasn't going anywhere.

The Crip Card refers to using this overly-nice treatment to your advantage. It is a membership card into the Crip Club, and like all exclusive clubs, it has its members-only benefits. As a member, your benefits package includes, but is not limited to: cutting lines without consequence, always having a good excuse to miss class, and exemption from security checks at sporting events and concerts.

After hearing several stories of the outrageous things people had gotten away with using the Crip Card—ditching class every Friday and still getting copies of the notes, bringing booze to football games because no one ever searches their bags—I felt emboldened to try it.

My friend from home had come to visit. We were supposed to go to the football game, but he had been unable to get a ticket. I told him with a mischievous smile, "It should be fine, we can still get you in." As we approached the gate, I gave him my ticket and told him to go first. Then I quickly zoomed in after him, without a ticket, and the person at the gate didn't say a word.

I couldn't believe it worked, and was quite proud of myself. Needless to say, this wouldn't be the last time I took advantage of the Crip Card.

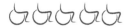

Aside from the terminology, this new language also had an alluring vulgarity to it. Political correctness was completely disregarded. Non-politically-correct terms like "cripple" and "gimp" were thrown around early and often. Someone might drop something on the floor and not be able to pick it up, and someone else would exclaim, "Man, you are so damn crippled!" I might hear someone say, "How does this shirt look on me? I don't want to look all gimpy."

The usual politically-correct language only seemed to be used in a facetious way. If someone were to fail at something that is usually considered effortless, like unwrapping tinfoil from a plate of leftovers, they might say with a sly grin, "I am handi-capable!" Whenever the "wrong" phrasing was used, no matter how harmlessly, it would still be corrected. For example, if a common saying like "flying blind" were to be used, someone might say, "No I think you mean 'flying with a visual impairment.'"

It was impressive how clever some of the jokes could be. We were all playing video games and I dropped my controller. I pled my case to stop the game, but that wasn't going to happen. Instead, someone took a common phrase absurdly out of context, "Don't use your disability as an excuse! You can pick it up; remember, you can do anything you put your mind to!" I wasn't even mad.

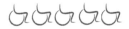

CULTURE SHOCK

PART TWO: STRANGE SOCIAL DYNAMIC

The Roberts language was certainly new and exciting, but it was nothing compared to what I stumbled upon next. I would soon encounter the real mind-blowing part of Roberts culture, what I have since come to call "Roberts-ism."

I witnessed it, one Friday night, as Phil and I were trying to watch a movie. The floater wasn't around to help, and we grew impatient. Phil said bitterly, "Forget it! I'll do it myself." I watched him get the disc out, loop his thumb through the hole in the middle, and slowly crawl his hand itsy-bitsy-spider style up the side of the TV, dragging his limp arm with it.

After several minutes of Phil struggling to put the disc in the DVD player, the floater and one of the live-in PAs entered the room. Instead of offering to help, they both cheered him on like he was chugging a beer, "GO! GO! GO!"

At first, I was too shocked to know how to react. I looked at the girls, then at Phil: they were all smiling. It was then that I realized this madness was serving as some sort of bonding ritual, as if we were all brought closer together by our lack of political correctness.

Something similar happened again, during lunch, a few days later. Only this time, the residents were doing it to a PA: a new girl doing her first meal assistant shift. She was visibly nervous, and a little unsure of how to act around so many people in wheelchairs.

Alan unknowingly initiated the ritual. He was making small talk to try and put her at ease, and asked the girl what she was doing later. She replied, "I'm probably going to go for a run later." That was all they needed; the older residents jumped at the opportunity. Someone said with a sly grin on their face, "That must be nice." Another one joined in from across the table: "What's that like?"

It was strange. I wondered, "Are they being assholes or not?" I honestly didn't know. I would have assumed calling out a new PA for talking about running would make them feel guilty or awkward, but this seemed to make her more comfortable.

They continued to make little comments for the rest of lunch, and after a while the new girl started smiling and laughing along with everyone.

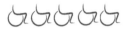

I was intrigued. I wasn't sure what I had been witnessing, but I knew it was a good thing. My peers seemed to have a means to alleviate disability-related awkwardness, and to top it off, it looked fun to do. I was waiting for my next opportunity.

It happened during my shower shift later in the week. My PA Anna accidentally stubbed my toe while lifting me, and I could tell she felt bad. So, I replied, "It's okay, I'm not going to be using it anytime soon." She laughed, and her grief instantly disappeared.

I thought to myself, "Wow! It worked." How exciting! Awkward situations didn't have to be a foregone conclusion anymore.

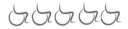

CULTURE SHOCK

PART THREE: TRUST

I had a Monday/Wednesday shower shift with Tom, for two consecutive school years. That's three hours a week for sixty-four weeks, which comes out to about two hundred hours spent together. Needless to say, we were homies by the end.

All of our shifts would follow the same routine: Tom would come in and tell me a story of some drunken adventure from the weekend, we would gossip about Roberts drama, there would be a shower in there somewhere, and, of course, the occasional heart-to-heart conversation.

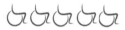

One day Tom came in and was noticeably extremely upset, which was strange because he never showed an ounce of vulnerability. I wasn't sure how to react, so I continued as usual. I started to tell him about some of the current Roberts drama, and when I got to the end of the story: nothing. Silence.

Tom wasn't paying any attention. He was staring blankly into the distance, doing the shift on autopilot. I thought, "This must be serious."

As I was lying there, having socks put on my feet, it was oppressively quiet. I was racking my brain, trying to figure out what I should do or say, when Tom began talking: "I'm not sure what I should do. I'm considering breaking up with my girlfriend."

I was shocked. This was one of those relationships that had been going strong since high school; they had been together for about five or six years. Tom and Vanessa did everything together. They lived together; their whole lives revolved around each other. It was always pretty much understood that they were inevitably going to get married. So, this was huge.

I asked, "What do you mean?" Tom sighed deeply, "I'm just not feeling it lately. The spark is gone. I already know everything about her, there's no real surprises anymore." "Maybe you—" I was cut off mid-sentence as Tom continued, "Lately I started going to the gym and I've been thinking, 'Why am I putting all this effort into staying fit and looking good for her when she is completely letting herself go?' I even hinted that she should start going with me. She's honestly starting to get a little fat, and I don't want to be married to a fat lady my whole life—especially when I am still putting in the work to look good."

I had no idea how to respond, "I honestly don't know what to tell you. I've never been in a long-term relationship, so I haven't really been in your situation." Then, Tom said something I will never forget: "Give me *something*, man. You're the only one I've told about this." I asked why, and he replied, "Because you're the only one I trust."

I had to fight the urge to get all sentimental and say,

"REALLY?!!" Luckily, I was able to keep cool. I replied with: "I certainly don't want to be blamed for telling you to end your relationship. All I'll say is you are still young and you are not locked in yet. If you were to end everything, now would be the time to do it. You're about to go to grad school in Arizona, and that's a good opportunity to start over. But, think long and hard before you do anything." This answer seemed to satisfy him, and he went back to staring into the distance. We finished the rest of the shift in silence.

This was the first time something like this had happened. After he left, I was astonished. Did he really trust me more than any of his other friends? After all, I only saw him two days a week.

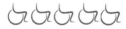

As time went on, I saw that it wasn't just Tom; a large majority of PAs really trusted me. Anna told me about all the behavioral issues her younger sister was having at school, another PA confessed to me that she had cheated on her boyfriend, not to mention the countless female PAs who would cry in front of me over the years.

I always wondered why PAs felt so comfortable around me, and I eventually figured it out. When you receive help with personal care, you have to open yourself up to people, allowing them to see you in your most private and intimate moments. In doing so, you are showing the other person that you really trust them. And, as time goes on, they are more inclined to trust you. You open yourself up to them, and they are more willing to open up to you.

Put another way: after they have seen me naked, and gotten up close and personal with my nether regions, I can't really judge. They have already seen me at my worst, so they have no reason to be embarrassed.

CHAPTER ELEVEN

LETTING LOOSE

Anyone who has gone away to college knows partying and drinking are a big part of the culture. This is especially true of freshmen. Given their newly acquired freedom, most freshmen party and let loose. They are free to make all of their own decisions—good and mostly bad. I too felt the allure of this culture, but I didn't get many opportunities to partake during my first year. I had more important things to attend to, see: the last three chapters.

Now, as I began my sophomore year, I was finally at the point where I had no more growing pains. My top priority shifted from learning what the hell I was doing to letting loose and having fun.

ᘒᘒᘒᘒᘒ

LETTING LOOSE

PART ONE: DIVING IN HEAD FIRST

I went out as soon as I could: the very first weekend of the school year. Alan, Ron, and I went to the Rogue Ales: the only bar we could get into; it was in the next town—where you only had to be eighteen to get into bars. I'm not sure how they were able to swing that, legally speaking, but I wasn't going to ask questions.

We arrived at the Rogue Ales, and I was so excited I could barely contain myself; I was actually in a real college bar! It was just like I imagined: deafening music, gorgeous women, and sloppy drunk people. I was in heaven.

The only thing that could have made it better was if we could actually buy some drinks. It may have been legal for us to enter, but we still had to be twenty-one to buy anything.

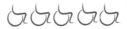

We were about to ask a stranger to go to the bar for us, when a familiar face approached. Enter Anna and her roommate—also a PA at Roberts.[25] A chance encounter with off-duty PAs was always exciting, especially when they were two pretty girls; made even better still when they were of-age and could buy us drinks.

They went to the bar, and later came back with five Long Island Iced Teas. And just when I thought this chance meeting couldn't get any better, Anna volunteered as my designated drinker for the night.[26]

---

25 They both knew each other outside of work. It wasn't uncommon that a group of friends would all start working as PAs at the same time.
26 A common wheelie problem is being unable to hold your own drink. When someone else holds it for you, we call that a "designated drinker."

I attempted to nurse my drink, still trying to be careful and find my limits gradually, but Anna was not making it easy. She kept holding the cup in front of my face until I took a drink, and each time I drank she would playfully insist I take just a tiny bit more. Whenever I refused, she would simply turn up the persistence until I gave in.

I did my best to resist her charms, but very quickly finished my drink. This concerned me because I had never finished an entire drink before. I wasn't sure how it would affect me.

After a while, I only felt a slight buzz, and was confident I could handle another one, as long as I was adamant about drinking it slow.

I asked Anna to go back to the bar, and she was happy to do so. But, by the time she returned, we were getting ready to leave. It was almost ten, and we were supposed to be at Tom's party.

I thanked Anna for getting me another Long Island, but politely declined: "I have to go. We're late for our friend's party." Anna replied, in a semi-flirty but aggressive tone, "No, I went and got it for you. You're finishing it! Just drink fast." She then proceeded to give me a puppy-dog face, bat her eyes and say, "Come on, please? You can do it," in a cutesy voice. And, just like that, I completely abandoned my vow to be careful with alcohol. I chugged the entire thing.

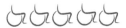

It took only a few minutes before I was bombarded with a flurry of new sensations: the warm fuzzy-in-the-face feeling, the way everything sort of slows down, the dulling of your awareness. I was amazed at seeing the world for the first time with drunk eyes.

Then, as soon as I started to move, my fascination turned into dread. Driving my wheelchair was suddenly a lot more difficult; with everything—accelerating, stopping, turning—the chair seemed to be moving faster than I could react. That, combined with avoiding the mobs of people, made getting out an ordeal. Navigating my wheelchair through the condensed crowd would have been hard enough if I were at full capacity, let alone drunk for the first time.

After what seemed like an eternity, I made it outside. I could finally breathe again. The cool air felt rejuvenating after being smothered by the collective body heat of a hundred strangers.

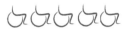

I was barely able to appreciate my escape from the bar before I encountered a new crisis. I immediately had a fierce urge to use the bathroom. No one had told me drinking made you have to pee so badly. I never got that memo and, with the girls still inside, I would have to hold it until we got to our next destination.[27]

As I was pondering the long and uncomfortable wait, Alan had meanwhile flagged down a bus. My friends were halfway down the street, preparing to board, by the time I focused my attention back to them. I yelled, "Wait for me!" and scurried as fast as my wheels could carry me.

The driver pulled up next to the curb, the ramp was deployed, and we all piled onto the bus. The accessible space on a city bus is a tight squeeze, especially with more than the regulation two wheelchairs crammed into it, but that didn't stop us from trying.

The way we arranged ourselves was a mess: completely blocking the aisle and forcing other riders to enter through the rear door; it was not befitting three experienced wheelchair-users.

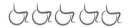

We arrived and before Tom even had the door halfway open, I was frantically pleading with him: "I have to use the bathroom! I have to go now!" Seeing the urgency in my face, he swung the door open and cleared a path to the bathroom, shoving people out of the way. With a lightning-

---

27 Another common wheelie problem is having to pee. If there is no one around to help, you simply have to wait.

fast efficiency I had never seen during an ordinary PA shift, Tom had me peeing in no less than three seconds.

As I exited the bathroom, I saw my two friends already had drinks and were mingling with Tom's friends. I made my way to Tom's roommate, who was passing out red cups. As I got closer, I could see he was actually using the cups to scoop a red liquid from a big orange Gatorade cooler. I asked what it was and he answered: "It's jungle juice. You want some?" "Sure, what's in it?" He explained as he scooped a cup for me, "A handle of vodka, half a bottle of apple juice, and about twenty Kool-Aid packets. Be careful, this stuff will fuck you up." I assured him I could handle it—I could not. None of us wheelies were prepared for this lethal concoction.

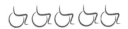

Tom's roommate dropped a straw in my cup and gave me a drink—it didn't taste nearly as awful as the recipe would suggest. He helped me for a few minutes, but was soon called to play beer pong and passed my drink along to the person next to him: "Here, Jackie can you help him?" Before she could even turn around, he was gone.

"Jackie" seemed a bit uncomfortable about the arrangement, but I was buzzed enough to not care. I ignored her discomfort, and proceeded to talk her ear off.

It was probably a bit obnoxious, but my incessant chatter did eventually put her at ease. After a while, she timidly said, "There has always been something I've wanted to ask someone in a wheelchair, but I was afraid it would be weird." I assured her it was fine, so Jackie went ahead and asked, "Why do people in wheelchairs wear shoes? You don't really need them." I thought about it for a minute and replied, "That never occurred to me before. I guess we don't really need shoes, but it's more socially acceptable to wear them."

This was the icebreaker I had been waiting for. Jackie's awkwardness disappeared after this little exchange and, from that point forward, the conversation came easy.

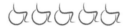

It was a really nice evening: our conversation was becoming more and more personal, and Jackie continued to feed me drinks, while I continued to graciously accept them. Everything was going great, until jungle juice claimed its first victim.

Ron was getting to a level of intoxication I hadn't yet known existed. He began constantly falling over and needing help to be uprighted. Ron had also lost any ability to effectively drive his wheelchair: he kept running over toes, and had a couple of near misses that could have seriously injured someone.

When Ron knocked over the beer pong table, it was the end of his night. Tom walked right over and disengaged his wheelchair;[28] then he proceeded to push Ron all the way back to the dorm.

After the spectacle of Ron leaving, I wondered how close I was to ending up like him. My body had been getting increasingly unhappy since I started drinking the jungle juice; I had a stomach full of spicy Asian food, and all the alcohol was not helping the situation. I knew it would have been wise to stop.

Nonetheless, Jackie got me another cup and for some reason—whether it be the alcohol affecting my judgment or the attention from a pretty girl—I couldn't say no. I stupidly continued.

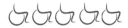

Jackie started to tell me about her life: she was really close with her family, she was from Iowa and went home to visit quite often, and she had recently broken up with her boyfriend—who still lived back home. My ears perked up at that last detail: "That's too bad. Maybe you just need to forget about him for a while." I thought I was so smooth.

Meanwhile, jungle juice claimed its second victim. Alan threw up in his cup, and Tom immediately took him into the bathroom. I should have been more concerned for my own welfare, considering Alan and Ron were experienced drinkers and I wasn't, but I was preoccupied. The only

---

28 The motor on a power wheelchair can be disengaged, allowing the chair to be pushed manually.

thing I cared about was keeping my conversation going as long as possible.

Jackie then asked, "Does it bother you when you can't do stuff?" I was thoroughly prepared to sound smart and thoughtful while I delivered my answer: "It used to, but I've learned to find value in other things—" I had to stop as I felt my stomach rumbling.

I continued, hoping I didn't throw up: "I've never really engaged in sports or other physical activities, so they are not really a part of my life—" I started dry-heaving and trying my damnedest to stifle down the vomit.

Jackie—bless her heart—mistook the dry-heaving for crying. She started patting me on the back and saying, "It's okay. Playing sports isn't important."

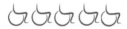

Not wanting to be the third victim, I immediately decided it was time to leave. I ended the conversation, as politely as I could, and got ready to go. I headed toward the door, as Alan was leaving the bathroom, and the two of us left together.

Then, as soon as we got downstairs, Alan inexplicably zoomed ahead, leaving me alone. I wasn't sure what was going on; I tried "flooring it" to catch him, but immediately had to slow down.

Driving over the less than stellar pavement of Wallace Street felt like being in one of those funhouse tunnels where the floor is tilting back and forth. Every little bump and imperfection in the street was dizzying. I slowed to a crawl-like pace; all the while, an intense urge to go to the bathroom was building.

The return home became a long and painful experience, but I eventually made it back. I turned the corner, toward the floater desk, and like Chevy Chase arriving at a closed Wally World, was devastated to see an empty chair. Another student was sitting in the lobby, and they informed me Alan was using the floater.

"That sneaky son of a bitch!" I hadn't realized the reason Alan was so eager to get back before me was so he could get to the floater first.

As I would learn, whenever the Roberts crowd comes back from a night out, there is always a rat race to get to the floater first. I was certainly going to be aware from that point forward.

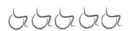

LETTING LOOSE

PART TWO: A HALLOWEEN ADVENTURE

Halloween was a special occasion at Roberts. Every year, our crew made a group costume that incorporated our wheelchairs. This was never an easy task but, for a few years, we managed to come up with some good ideas:

Mario Kart, a biker gang, and—my personal favorite—the Jamaican bobsled team from the movie *Cool Runnings*. We all had matching jumpsuits and made each of our wheelchairs look like part of the bobsled; driving the four of our chairs in single file completed the look.

The following story takes place during the Mario Kart Halloween. Ron was Mario, I was Luigi, and Alan was Yoshi.

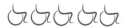

The night began ordinarily enough: another party at Tom's apartment, copious amounts of alcohol, and plenty of bad decisions to go around. It was pretty much business as usual for a Saturday night, until we left to go to the bars.

On the way out of Tom's place, there was a group of students playing live music on the corner. Without explanation, one of Tom's friends—who played the guitar himself—took the guitar from the lead singer, and began to play.

Surprisingly, the band just improvised along with him. And, even more surprisingly, Ron and Tom started singing too.

At that point, it hit me that something really cool was happening. However, I couldn't enjoy the special moment for long because Alan had passed out in his chair, and I was the only one who noticed.

I frantically tried to get the attention of our able-bodied

friends, but they continued singing, blissfully unaware of the urgent situation. "We're almost done with this song. It's *Wonderwall*, we have to finish," was the answer I got.

As soon as the "beautiful" cover of *Wonderwall* was over, they saw Alan and all ran over.

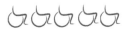

It was clear Alan needed to get home as quickly as possible. Though getting him there wasn't going to be easy. It took three people to get him down the street: one to hold his head up, one to navigate, and a third one to push the wheelchair.

In ten minutes, they had only managed to move a few blocks, and it became clear the current strategy wasn't going to work. At that pace, it would have taken an hour to get him back. Tom made the executive decision to just drive Alan back to the dorm, and left to go get his car.

After a short while, Tom pulled up in his old rusty sedan. Anna picked Alan up and laid him across the back seat; she would stay in the back with him while Tom drove.

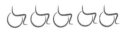

Meanwhile, Tom's friend, dressed as the Pillsbury dough-boy, drove Alan's wheelchair. I don't mean that he disengaged the brakes and pushed it; he actually sat in the wheelchair and drove it.

I couldn't stop laughing at how ridiculous the situation was: he was obviously too big, and not meant to be sitting in that chair. The humor wasn't lost on him either. He zoomed ahead of us, pointed forward, and yelled: "Let's move out boys!"

Our wheelchair convoy of the Pillsbury doughboy, Mario, and Luigi, headed toward the bar. It probably would've been wise to return to the dorm, and get Alan's wheelchair back to his room, but we weren't going to let the loss of a comrade ruin our night.

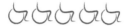

Then I must have blacked out because, all of a sudden, it was morning. The first thing I realized, upon waking up, was that I was not in my room—I had no idea where I was. I also didn't have my phone, and I couldn't just get up and run out of there either. Once it dawned on me that I was trapped in this place, I started to panic.

After several minutes of silently freaking out, my morning grogginess subsided, and I calmed down enough to start looking around. I was lying on a dirty gray couch, facing a plain white wall with nothing on it but a singular poster of Lil' Wayne: shirtless with saggy pants, his metallic teeth shining bright against a pot-leaf backdrop. I strained my neck to see behind me, and noticed a TV with equal parts pizza grease and SportsCenter on the screen, with a Nintendo 64 on the floor in front of it. With that last detail,

I was certain of where I was—I only knew one person with a Nintendo 64. I wondered, "How on earth did I end up at Tom's apartment?"

I called out for Tom several times, and then felt something stirring on the floor next to the couch; I was very relieved when I saw it was Anna, and told her as much. She helped me get in my wheelchair, and walked back to Roberts with me.

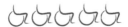

As I entered the front door of the dorm, my PA was also walking in for his regularly scheduled shift to get me out of bed for the day. He looked at me with a very confused expression. Then he looked at the floater, and she told him I had just gotten home after being out all night.

My PA looked at me like he wanted to know the story, and I returned a look that said I barely slept and still felt slightly drunk. He immediately understood that I needed to get in bed as soon as possible.

We proceeded to do the usual routine in reverse order. The shift was quickly finished, and, as soon as my head hit the pillow, I was out cold.

CHAPTER TWELVE

THERE'S A FIRST TIME FOR EVERYTHING

Alan, Ron, and I all headed out to The Summit, with Tom and his roommates, as we did every Friday night. It was usually a pretty chill time but, every once in a while, there was a big crowd. On this particular night, the Summit was packed; the crowd was so raucous we could barely hear each other.

The table next to us was especially loud, engaged in an intense game of flippy-cup. "Who plays a drinking game in a bar?!" I was getting annoyed with their noise level, and I couldn't wait for them to leave.

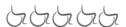

Eventually the flippy-cup game ended, and the table cleared out. All of them left, except for one. A girl stayed around, and started drooling over Tom: being blatantly flirtatious, and physically affectionate. He was a pretty good-looking dude, and occurrences like this were not all that uncommon.

Typically, Tom would completely shut them down, they

would give up and leave, and then we would continue where we left off. Only this time, the girl didn't leave.

She must have been on the prowl for any male attention, because she instantly turned her focus to me.

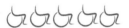

My new friend asked if I wanted to dance, and I awkwardly accepted. I wasn't sure how that was going to go, considering I can barely move my body. But I did my best to keep her engaged—smiling, moving my head and arms as much as I could—and it seemed to work: she stayed around for a few songs.

Then she abruptly left. And I assumed that was the end; this girl had experienced the novelty of dancing with a wheelie, and now she had moved on to bigger and better things. But my assumption couldn't have been more wrong.

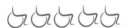

After ten minutes, she came back with a drink in her hand. Pulling a chair next to me, she introduced herself as Madison. This had never happened before. How peculiar. Madison then apologized for leaving. Doubly peculiar. And when she asked if I wanted to share her drink, I had to pinch myself.

As we shared her Jack and Coke, we proceeded to exchange playful drunk banter. I would react overly dramatically to something she said. She would tease me about something funny I did. Then we would start the interaction again, and each time we repeated the cycle, I enjoyed it more than the last.

It was all really exciting but, after we finished her drink, she went out for a smoke. I had been waiting for a sign that the situation wasn't what it looked like, and "going out to smoke" was probably it.

Everything I knew from past experience told me she wasn't coming back. Wheelies just didn't pick up girls at bars. Kissing a girl or two, and even dating a PA, were in the realm of possibility, but bringing home a stranger from a bar was unheard of at Roberts.

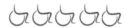

Then, to my astonishment, Madison returned with another drink. "Is this really happening? A girl like this couldn't be interested in someone like me, could she?"

As I was still grappling with my insecurities, Tom diagnosed the situation and decided it was time for everyone else to leave. He promptly took Alan and Ron home.

After this savvy act of wingmanship, I knew I wasn't just imagining things. I started to believe.

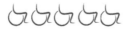

Over the next hour, the situation escalated. The teasing

started to be interspersed with really personal conversation, the eye contact was more frequent and lasted longer, and the physical affection intensified. All the while, I could tell Madison was waiting for me to do something, but I wasn't sure what. I knew I needed to make a move, but I honestly had no idea what that looked like. What was the right time? Did I just ask directly, or was it supposed to be more subtle?

As I contemplated what to do, all the lights came on. A voice announced that the bar was closing, and I knew it was now or never. I took a deep breath, and very simply let Madison know I didn't want her to leave. She replied, "I would love to stay, but I don't go to this school, I'm just visiting. I have to meet up with my friends or I'll get lost."

After telling me the address, she asked if I knew where her friend's place was; I assured her I knew. I said something to the effect of: "I'll show you where that is, after I show you where I live." I still have absolutely no idea where that line came from, but it worked: Madison decided to come home with me.

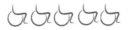

Madison climbed up on my lap, wanting me to be her wheelie chauffeur. I eagerly accepted the job, though without giving much thought to how that would work. I hadn't realized having someone sit on my lap would obstruct both my view and my grasp on the controller.[29] It was all I could do to simply maintain control.

Despite nearly running into a parked car, we both made it safely back to Roberts. Madison rang the doorbell,[30] and the RA answered the door. He instantly knew what was going on, and seemed as excited about what was happening as I was.

The RA basically escorted us to my room. Madison and I both followed him and, as we entered the room, he closed the door behind us.

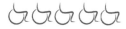

As it hit me that this was actually going to happen, my nervousness amplified tenfold. I had never kissed a girl before, let alone brought one home. I had no idea what I was supposed to do or say, or how the logistics of the situation would work.

Luckily, I didn't have to worry for long. Before I had a chance to freak out, she leaned in and kissed me. I didn't know the best way to position my wheelchair, so we were both awkwardly hunched forward, but I was perfectly fine with that.

I was trying my best to mimic whatever she did and I was holding my own—all things considered. Then, as we started to get into it, a terrible thought popped into my

---

29 The joystick controller that drives a power wheelchair.
30 The front doors locked after midnight.

head: "How long can I keep this up before I do something completely wrong and blow it?"

I certainly didn't want to embarrass myself in front of this gorgeous girl, who was actually into me. I decided to quit while I was ahead, and ended it.

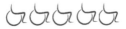

We both headed toward the main entrance, as Madison prepared to leave. I should have seen her out, but I was too drunkenly excited to remember my manners. Instead of giving Madison the directions to her friend's house I had promised, I zoomed to the computer lab to tell everyone.

She ended up asking the RA for directions to her friend's place. This wasn't my classiest moment, but at least I could now say I kissed a girl.

CHAPTER THIRTEEN

A BITTERSWEET FAREWELL

Returning from winter break, there was a freak blizzard. The interstate was covered in a dangerous amount of snow; and traffic was moving at about thirty miles per hour.

None of the streets were plowed when we drove into town, and the sidewalks still needed to be cleared.

Finding a place to deploy the wheelchair lift was going to be a struggle in itself, let alone driving my wheelchair through the literal inches of snow.

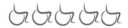

This weather always made me nervous because snow can be quite the hazard for wheelchairs. I had, on more than one occasion, gotten stuck in unshoveled curb cuts, slid off the sidewalk, and lost traction going down the ramp in my backyard.

Then, after crunching my way through the freshly powdered sidewalks, my fears were realized. As I attempted to get up the ramp in front of the building, I lost traction and slid back down. In order to make it up, my dad and a random good Samaritan had to stand behind my wheelchair and push.

It took a while, but I finally made it to flat ground. As I passed through the double doors and heard my snow-covered wheels squeaking against the linoleum floor, I let out a big sigh of relief.

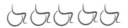

I was able to breathe easy, having made it through the latest snowfall without incident. However, I would soon learn not everyone had been so lucky. That evening, I received an ominous text message from Anna: "What's wrong with Phil? It sounds serious."

I was sorry to say that I didn't know. We had sort of fallen out of touch after Phil moved out of Roberts.

A few days later, Anna informed me he had been rushed to the hospital, and was still in intensive care. Upon hearing this, I immediately called Phil to see if everything was okay, and received no answer.

The next morning, Anna came to my room to tell me Phil had passed away. And, I don't know if we were in shock or just didn't know what to say, but we both sat in silence until she left.

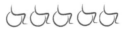

Alan, Ron, and I, did not go to class that day. Instead, we

went to one of the common study areas, and didn't leave for several hours. We all shared stories about Phil, and vented about how we felt. It was very therapeutic.

We were later joined by Tom and Anna. Tom had spoken with Phil's mother on the phone, and was able to give us the details of what had happened.

It had occurred Sunday, during the snowstorm. One of the ramps, leading into his dorm, had been especially slippery with all the snow. And, at some point during his descent, Phil lost control of his wheelchair; it tipped over, causing him to fall out.

As a result of the fall, Phil broke both of his femurs and his pelvis; his bones were especially brittle due to the steroid regimen he had been on. He was so severely injured that he had to be airlifted to a hospital ninety miles away.

Phil put up a good fight, but the internal injuries he sustained proved to be too much for his system. He passed away three days later.

It was not easy to hear the details of a friend's death, but I think it was something we all needed to know.

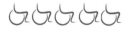

The service was the upcoming weekend, which was really short notice for all of us. It would normally take about a week or two to make the travel arrangements for a long-distance drive; but given the importance of the situation, we rallied together and got it done within a day.

Ron immediately offered his accessible van, which his mom then drove for two hours to bring to us. We needed a driver, and Anna volunteered without us having to ask. Then, the three of us each needed our own PA to travel with, and we all found someone.

I was actually surprised with how painless the planning had been—all things considered. Everyone had been eager to help us. I guess they knew how important it was that we be there.

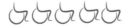

Later, when the Catholic church on campus hosted a memorial mass for Phil and his family, it was more of the same. Everyone from Roberts went: our entire friend group, several PAs, staff, and even some of the new residents who never personally knew Phil.

That entire week, I had been both impressed and over-joyed with the way the entire community rallied around this tragedy. I know it is only a small consolation, but it seemed that Phil's passing had brought the community closer together.

CHAPTER FOURTEEN

UNABLE TO COPE

We all coped with the grief differently. Ron and Alan started going out and drinking way more than usual. Whereas, I just wanted to be alone, spending a lot of time by myself.

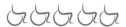

It was a weeknight, and it played out the same way every night had played out since the memorial: Alan and Ron had gone out, and I chose not to join them.

I was watching a movie in my room, when I received a phone call. It was Ron asking me to come to The Lotus— their favorite Chinese restaurant, and favorite stop after a night out.

I declined, but Ron insisted it was an emergency: Alan was having a bad night. I knew Alan had taken Phil's passing the hardest, so I ultimately agreed to meet them.

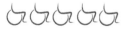

As I approached The Lotus, I could see, through its sidewalk-facing window. Alan's head was flat on the table.

He was noticeably upset, and appeared to be saying something. And when I entered, I could see Ron was sitting across from Alan, trying to reason with him.

Before I could say anything, Ron immediately started debriefing me: "One minute he was fine, and then he threw up. He fell on the table and started yelling about how his friend was taken away. And, 'It could have happened to any of us!'"

He was frantically telling me that Alan needed his friends right now, and he needed to confront his grief, and on and on. But, being the only sober one, I could easily see that all Alan really needed was to get home.

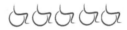

As Ron and I argued over the best course of action, Alan suddenly sat up. He looked at us for a second, and then fell backward against the back of his wheelchair, his head perpendicular to the back of the seat.

Then he began to throw up in his mouth, but was too drunk to lift his head back up. This is when the situation turned dangerous: if he didn't get his head lifted up soon, he was going to choke.

I couldn't physically help Alan, and Ron was trying his best but couldn't manage on his own. And, to make matters worse, there was no one else in the place we could ask for help.

Then I remembered that there was one guy at the

counter. I zoomed over to the guy, and explained the situation. All he did was smile and nod. I assumed he didn't quite understand what I was saying, and repeated myself. Again, he smiled and nodded, and did nothing.

I was really confused for a second, and then it dawned on me: this man doesn't speak English. All I could do was try to motion his attention to Alan. One look at him and this guy would know what was wrong. But he just wasn't understanding.

In a panic, I yelled over to Ron: "Dude! This guy doesn't understand what I'm saying!" He rushed over and pointed in the direction of Alan. The guy peeked out over the counter, and I could see the look of instant recognition on his face. He immediately turned and ran through the kitchen and out to the dining area, with a Styrofoam take-home box in his hand. He lifted Alan's head up, and used the box to help him finish throwing up.

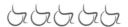

We both breathed a sigh of relief, knowing our friend was no longer in mortal danger. But we were so spooked by the situation that we decided to call an ambulance.

After ten minutes passed, the EMTs arrived. The one in charge took a look at Alan, and told us he would be fine; we just needed to get someone to bring him home.

I called Tom, and he came right over. I brought him up

to speed, and he proceeded to push Alan all the way back to the dorm.

The whole way back, I could tell Tom was not happy. I repeatedly apologized, and assured him he wouldn't have to take care of Alan when we got back—that was the RA's job.

After a long and difficult trek, we finally made it back. Alan was immediately handed off to the RA, and the crisis was over.

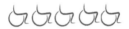

My nerves were fried. As Anna got me ready for bed, I was a mess. I ended up unloading on her: the stress from Alan's ordeal, as well as unresolved grief from Phil's passing, all came pouring out. Anna listened patiently, and stayed with me until I calmed down.

CHAPTER FIFTEEN

A MUCH-NEEDED ESCAPE

This most recent incident made it painfully clear that the three of us were not handling Phil's passing very well. After seeing Alan, a drunken mess, and experiencing my own emotional freak out, I decided it was time for a much-needed escape. And when I discussed it with Alan and Ron, they both felt the same way.

We needed a vacation, a chance to relax and blow off some steam. Alan, Ron, and I, had been dealing with losing a close friend for several months, and it was time to recharge.

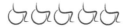

We were young college students, so we naturally decided on the vacation every college kid wants: spring break.

My only concern with the idea was whether it was in poor taste. Was going on a big debauchery-filled vacation, so soon after Phil's passing, disrespectful to his memory?

I was unsure about the whole thing, but then Ron— who has a knack for saying profound things at the perfect moment—put my mind at ease: "We can't mourn forever.

Part of grieving is finding a way to keep on living your life. And besides, Phil wouldn't have wanted us to stop having fun."

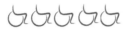

A MUCH-NEEDED ESCAPE

PART ONE: PLANNING

The spring break trip was officially moving forward, and I was so excited by the idea that I took the lead in planning it.

I made a list of everything that needed to be figured out, and it was massive. But, as someone with a severe disability, I am no stranger to meticulous planning. I immediately got to it.

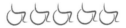

The first issue to deal with was coordinating PAs. This would be difficult, because we had to: find people willing to go, compensate them for helping us, and then spend the additional money to pay for their travel and lodging.

The next item to tackle was the location. Wheelies cannot easily go to every popular vacation destination, so I needed to make sure the place we chose was accessible.

Anywhere without spacious hotel rooms or smooth paved ground was a definite no-go.

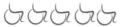

We had initially wanted to go to Las Vegas but, after looking into it, the idea didn't seem feasible.

For one, it was far, and I was not so keen on flying—airline baggage workers are notorious for breaking wheelchairs. But my fears aside, the airfare was also outrageous—especially considering we would be paying for our PAs.

As an alternative, I looked into taking a train, but that wasn't going to work either. The closest station was nearly thirty miles away from the city.

I didn't want to give up on Las Vegas, but the train was our last option. I unfortunately had to close the book on that idea—it was just not going to work.

Our second choice was New Orleans, and it was clearly the better option. It was closer, less expensive, the train station was actually in the city, and, of course, New Orleans was equally as famous for being "morally gray."

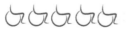

After a few weeks, the big hurdles were cleared. The PAs were scheduled—Anna and Tom, we had our location, and

I booked an accessible yet affordable hotel. Now it was time to address the logistics.

Our preferred mode of transportation was train, but it too was not without its problems. All of the long-distance tickets were overnight, which would require sleeping on the train. And I wasn't sure how that was going to go: Alan and I can't sleep while sitting up.

Then I noticed one of the routes had those sleeping cars with the beds. They were quite a bit more expensive than the regular coach seats—but it was either that or go without sleep. So, I said "RIP" to my wallet, and bought the Amtrak tickets: three coach—Ron would sleep in his wheelchair in the coach car—and two sleepers.

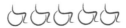

Then there was the issue of our medical equipment. The list of things we needed to bring was also pretty lengthy: medical devices, shower chairs, a lot of specialized pillows, and on and on; we couldn't possibly take it all.

The three of us needed to downsize, and only bring what was absolutely necessary. I decided I could go without my supplemental tube feedings; that would be six cartons of formula and the feed pump scratched off the list. Alan also decided to lighten the load, and make do with just the pillows at the hotel, leaving his orthotic pillows at home.

Then we talked it over, and decided to share my shower chair[31]—kind of gross, but we did what we had to do.

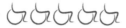

Before I knew it, the planning deadline had crept up on me. It was the big day: we were leaving for New Orleans.

As we boarded, the plan seemed to be going smoothly. One of the workers brought out the big hydraulic lift, and hoisted Ron up into a coach car at the front of the train. He and Anna both got settled, while the rest of us were directed toward our sleeper car at the back of the train.

Alan was the next to be lifted, and then it was my turn to use the rickety hand-cranked machine. While I was incrementally jolted upward with each pull of the lever, I saw Tom take the power strip from my bag, preparing to plug in the wheelchair chargers.

The need for a lot of outlets was a detail I had made a point of remembering. I was quite proud of myself.

Though this feeling didn't last long. We immediately ran into a problem, and had to start improvising. The sleeper car was too small to fit two wheelchairs. The beds took up majority of the space in the room; other than that, there was only a tiny walkway, and it was a tight fit for a wheelchair. Tom had to partially take my chair apart just so he could get it in the room.

Alan's wheelchair, on the other hand, was left outside

---

31 A water-proof wheelchair used in the shower. It also goes over the toilet.

the door. This was a huge inconvenience for the other passengers, who had to squeeze past Alan's chair to get to the bathroom. On top of that, there was also my shower chair, which we left in the foyer where passengers board and unboard.

These things may have been inconsiderate, but we did what we had to do. Sometimes when you have a severe disability, you don't have the luxury of caring what other people think; there are times when everything goes wrong, and you just have to throw together a solution as quickly as possible.

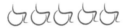

Despite a few hurdles on the train, we arrived in one piece. When we exited the train, the temperature was in the mid-seventies—in stark contrast to the mid-thirties we left behind. As my back was warmed by the heat of the tropical sun, I felt a strong wave of satisfaction come rushing through me.

It was not an easy thing to plan a trip for three people, with disabilities as severe as ours, but I had been able to make it work.

Then we left the station, and I realized I wasn't home-free just yet. To my horror, the area was absurdly inaccessible. What I had not realized is the train station, as well as our hotel, were in the oldest section of New Orleans. Some of the streets were cobblestone, others didn't have curb cuts, and the sidewalks seemed more appropriate for skilled rock climbers than pedestrians.

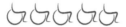

We made the trek through the urban jungle, carrying our luggage and medical equipment as we went. It must've been a sight to see our squad rolling down the street: three wheelchair users, two PAs, each carrying about fifteen pounds of luggage, and one of them also tugging along my shower chair—which had, resting on top, a white garbage bag overstuffed with specialized pillows. I thought to myself, as we passed each onlooker: "Excuse me, *National Lampoon's Wheelchair Vacation* coming through."

We eventually made it to the hotel, grabbed something to eat, and crashed. After the eighteen-hour train ride and journey to the hotel, all five of us were exhausted.

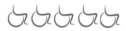

A MUCH-NEEDED ESCAPE

PART TWO: THE BIG EASY

After some much-needed rest, we were ready to head out on the town. Though, after seeing the condition of the sidewalks, I was not too keen on the walk from the hotel to Bourbon Street. Fortunately, Tom did some research and found that the New Orleans mass transit had a paratransit service.[32]

We scheduled a ride to take us to Bourbon Street, and the accessible bus arrived on schedule. We were greeted by a rather unkempt, slow-moving driver who smelled like weed. Ron whispered facetiously to me: "Even the bus drivers know how to party in New Orleans!" I laughed and replied, "It's not called The Big Easy for nothing."

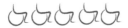

Naturally, the first thing we did, when we got to Bourbon Street, was get drinks. I spied a bar with a sign in the window: "Strongest Drink in the World." I decided to try it, and Anna retrieved one for me; the world's strongest drink turned out to be an alcoholic smoothie in a thin, four-foot-long novelty cup.

I took one sip and quickly realized that the world's strongest drink is not meant for human consumption. It was like drinking gasoline. Fortunately, I was able to quickly get another drink and remedy the situation.

Then, after exploring and sampling more of the local fare, the time had come. Being the gentlemen we are, it was only appropriate to pay a visit to the finest gentlemen's club we could find. The destination was the Penthouse Club, and I knew this place would be great before I even

32 Accessible vans that provide cheap, door-to-door rides to people with disabilities.

got inside. The bouncer was wearing a tux, and the main lobby had marble arches and a crystal chandelier.

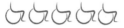

The next day promised to be an exciting one. Not only was it the last day of Mardi Gras; it was also St. Patrick's Day.

The first stop was a Mardi Gras parade, which Tom had found on the internet. It seemed a bit weird that none of us had ever heard of this particular parade, but he seemed confident so we just took his word for it.

The four of us followed Tom, who assured us he knew where to go. But, after a while, I started to have my doubts. We ventured farther and farther from the French Quarter, and eventually ended up in an area that was, shall we say, not in the brochure.

There were vacant lots everywhere, old condemned buildings that were starting to fall apart, barbed wire and steel gates adorned just about every place of business, and we passed probably three or four little roadside memorials—with lit candles and a picture of a young man's face—paying respects to different victims of gun violence. I'm not going to lie; I felt a little uneasy.

Then, to top things off, we passed a homeless man that was muttering to himself. As soon as he saw the wheelchairs, he got an unsettling wide-eyed look in his face. He started following us and asking questions about our disabilities. Alan and I were able to ignore him, but Ron had a bit of a panic attack, shouting: "I need to get out of here! I need to get back to the hotel!"

Tom stepped in and asked the homeless man to leave—which he did with no incident. And then we were able to calm Ron down, but only after our new friend was completely out of sight.

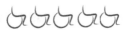

We eventually found the actual site of the parade, and I was relieved to see it was in a nicer area. And, upon seeing the direction of the flow of people to the area, it was clear we had not taken the intended route. The four of us had some choice words for Tom, and *politely* suggested that we take an alternative route back to the hotel.

We followed the crowd and found a nice spot to watch the parade. Once we were settled, I looked around and realized something was wrong. I was expecting a giant party, with constant beads and women flashing, but it was just an ordinary residential street. There were a few people camped out, in front of their houses, with coolers and food, but, other than that, there was no sign of festivities.

I was disappointed, and considering going back to the hotel—until the parade started passing by. The spectacle may not have been what I was expecting, but it still turned out to be really cool. The whole scene was exactly what you would think a parade in the Big Easy would be: people in feather-trimmed colorful costumes, voodoo imagery, dancing, and a lot of pageantry. You could almost hear the song *When the Saints Go Marching In* playing in the background.

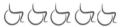

Before I knew it, the parade had all passed, and we were getting ready to head back to the hotel—taking the proper route this time. But before we left, I had to go to the bathroom; I had enjoyed one too many spirits, and it absolutely could not wait.

This was a problem because there were no Porta Potties anywhere, nor were there any buildings around that were even remotely accessible. So, just like with the train, I did what I had to do.

Tom and I snuck off to one of the side streets, which was deserted due to the parade, and desperately looked for an appropriate area where I could do my business. The best idea we could come up with was using the urinal in between two parked cars. At least then I would not be out in the open, visibility would be somewhat limited.

I started going, and not even ten seconds had passed, before a big crowd of people walked by. We both did our best to ignore them, but the drunk twenty-somethings were not being very subtle. A few of them shouted out whatever came to mind: "Whoa! What's going on there!" "Oh my God! What are they doing? Get a room!" All I can say is

I am glad I was somewhat tipsy, or that would have been really embarrassing.

After my bathroom ordeal, we went back and I headed straight to bed for a nap. I needed to rejuvenate if I was to be ready to go back out at night. We had another parade to attend—it was St. Patrick's Day after all.

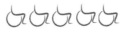

The paratransit bus dropped us off fairly early, so we were again able to find a great parade watching spot.

When the parade actually began, it was unlike anything I had ever seen. And I am no stranger to parties and debauchery either: I have been to St. Patrick's Day parades in Chicago. They looked tame compared to the New Orleans version.

All of the floats had bars on them, facing the crowd. Every so often, each float would stop and play a few songs while people went and bought drinks. It was essentially like barhopping, except each bar came to you.

After seeing how uninhibited the parade atmosphere was—and after a decent amount of adult beverages—our crew felt emboldened to join the parade. We just left our spot on the side of the street, and followed behind the bagpipers. We played along, waving and smiling at the crowd, and the funny thing was no one stopped us.

With three people in power wheelchairs, we could

have been representing some sort of disability or hospital organization; no one knew the difference.

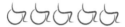

We eventually made it to the end of the parade route, and were all starving. Ron really wanted to get some authentic New Orleans seafood, and everyone agreed with the idea except for me. I personally hate that stuff, but I was outnumbered. We ended up going to the restaurant with the big banner outside saying it had fresh oysters and crawfish.

It certainly smelled "fresh." I couldn't get out of that place fast enough, and called the paratransit bus before the check came.

We returned to the hotel, and I was done. I went straight to bed, satisfied from the full and exciting day I had just experienced.

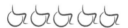

Just like that, our vacation was over. The five of us headed home the next morning. As we again boarded the train for the return ride, I was exhausted. Lying down in the sleeper car was pure bliss. And as I drifted to sleep, I felt a wave of satisfaction wash over me. The trip had been amazing, and I had planned everything pretty damn well too. To top things off, I no longer felt like a neurotic, stressed-out mess, and neither did Alan or Ron.

My last thought before passing out was: "mission accomplished." After that, I pretty much slept the entire sixteen-hour ride back home.

CHAPTER SIXTEEN

THE DATING GAME

PART ONE: GETTING MY FEET WET

From the beginning, Anna and I just clicked. I don't know if it was chemistry, or just having compatible personalities, but we became close right away. We had inside jokes, secrets, and all the other "best-friend stuff."

During our PA shifts, we talked about everything and anything. I found myself sharing personal things with her that I had never expected to tell anyone. I told her about my future dreams and aspirations, and even things that made me feel vulnerable, like: my fears or times that I cried.

We would sometimes take turns answering "big questions," and I couldn't believe the answers I would give.

Anna may have asked something like: "If you had unlimited resources, what would you do to change the world?" I was completely unafraid to say: "I would start my own airline that is completely wheelchair accessible." Another question might be: "What would be the ideal way to spend the rest of your life?" I had no problem admitting: "I can imagine living in a beachfront house in the Caribbean, selling food out of a truck part-time, making just enough money to live on."

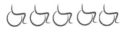

Anna and I also hung out a lot outside of work, watching *The Simpsons* or college basketball. We even had our own weekly routine.

Anna and I would go to the Women's Resource Center every Monday. They had speakers talk about women's issues, and offered free lunch to everyone that attended. It was meant to spread awareness and such, but we mostly just went for the food. We would simply ignore the presentation, and eat in the back of the room; without the distraction of the speaker, it was essentially the same as going out to lunch, only it was free.

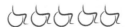

Then the inevitable happened. I was hit hard by the love bug. Anna became all I could think about.

She was funny, clever, beautiful, kind, and constantly looking for new experiences to better herself. Not to mention, she was in engineering—I'm a real sucker for smart girls.

We both had the same silly sense of humor, and a shared interest in all GMU sports—even the obscure ones. The list went on and on.

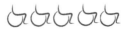

After months of secretly being in love with Anna, I decided to tell her how I felt. I had never asked a girl out before, and didn't really know what to do, but I didn't care. I needed to know if she felt the same way.

I had planned on saying something right away, but it ended up being way harder than I thought. Every time I planned on saying something, I would talk myself out of it. I would get nervous and find a reason not to go through with it.

I tried every approach I could to muster enough courage. I tried committing to it ahead of time, telling her, before she came over, that I wanted to talk. I tried setting a deadline for myself: "You will talk to Anna by the end of the month, just wait for the right time." But no time ever seemed right. It was one failure after another.

As I started to get desperate, I conjured an over-the-top scheme to create a romantic situation. I invited her to go listen to a real-life exorcist discuss his experiences, which was not the most romantic, but I only cared about after. We would walk home together, on the quad, and maybe the moon would be big and bright that night—it was perfect. There was no way it could fail.

Everything was going according to plan, but then, at the last minute, Anna invited her roommate to join. I was seriously frustrated at this point. I had to figure something out, because what I was doing was not working.

I decided I wouldn't do anything else until I had every detail figured out. How would I do it? Where? How could

I ensure I wouldn't chicken out? Would it be awkward? Would we still be friends afterwards? There was also the fact that she worked for me as a PA. Roberts had explicit rules against being romantically involved with a PA.

I tried my best to fit all the pieces together, but after a month or so, I still had no idea what to do. It was clear I would never have every detail figured out, no plan would be perfect, and no time would feel right. I just had to go for it.

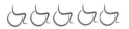

I was physically sick the entire day. All I could do, until Anna showed up, was continually rehearse what I was going to say.

After her shift was over, I offered to walk Anna home. I felt like throwing up as we approached her dorm, but I somehow managed to get all the words out. It was something along the lines of: "Anna, I like you more than a friend. And I was wondering if maybe you felt the same way?"

She respectfully informed me she did not feel the same way. So, sadly I did not get the answer I was hoping for, but, at least, I didn't lose my cool. Even though I was massively disappointed, I was able to end the interaction with dignity.

I was honestly surprised at how painless it was. I don't know what I was expecting—hostility, awkwardness, crying—but nothing bad happened. There were no hard feelings moving forward. In fact, we continued being close friends.

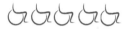

THE DATING GAME

PART TWO: DISAPPOINTMENT AND UNCERTAINTY

From the outside looking in, my recent introduction to the dating game had been a big success: I proved I had the courage to ask a girl out if I so choose, I handled the interaction with class, and my relationship with Anna was completely unharmed. I should've been satisfied, but I wasn't.

When I thought about what I would do differently with the next girl, I realized there probably wouldn't be a next girl. I knew dating is more difficult for people with disabilities, and my chances of finding someone else were not great.

Where exactly was I supposed to find someone? It certainly wasn't going to be in a class or at a party—most people were weird about the wheelchair when I first met them. If I approached a girl, at a party or something, there was a good chance she would smile awkwardly while wondering: "Is this disabled person actually trying to chat me up?" There would be a big wall of stereotypes to break through.

PA shifts, on the other hand, allowed for a lot of one-on-one time, a lot of time to break through some of those initial prejudices and stereotypes. In that regard, PAs seemed like the better way to go, but it would have been really creepy to actively seek that out. It was one thing if it just happened—a romantic connection with a PA—but I couldn't make that the goal. And even if I did, it was still no guarantee.

The more I thought about it, I was convinced I wouldn't find someone else. I just didn't see it happening. For a few weeks there, I went through a mini-depression. I started to constantly feel sorry for myself: "That's it. I'll never have a girlfriend." "People like me don't do that." I spent more time than I would like to admit listening to Coldplay alone in the dark.

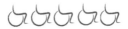

My melancholy was intense; I really felt hopeless about the situation. But luckily, that little funk didn't last long. It disappeared as I gradually witnessed things that contradicted my assumptions.

I had assumed the close connection I had with Anna was unique, but it turned out to be just the first of many. As I got better at being open, with my thoughts and feelings, close connections became commonplace. I grew close with many girls, PAs, and residents. My relationship with Anna became nothing special.

I had also assumed that dating was an extremely rare

occurrence for people with disabilities. But pretty soon several residents were in relationships. Alan started seeing a girl he met in class, another resident was dating one of the live-in PAs, and one guy eventually got engaged. I was both happy for everyone, and a little jealous at the same time.

Then there was the assumption that I could never find someone else. Of course, that ended up being wrong as well. I had plenty of opportunities, some that went well and far more that did not.

In short: I had been wrong. Dating turned out to be not nearly as impossible as I had thought.

ᕙᕙᕙᕙᕙ

THE DATING GAME

PART THREE: THE SEMIFORMAL

The idea of a date event had been thrown around Roberts for a while. Then, one year, the Roberts Student Council actually started planning a semiformal.

I was all for the idea; it was a long time coming. I had always thought we should be able to have the same sorts of social events as anyone else.

ᕙᕙᕙᕙᕙ

I was excited to begin thinking about who I would ask: making a mental list of girls I liked, and deciding who would be open to the idea.

Asking people out was no less scary this time, and I dragged my feet for weeks before settling on asking Anna. There was no pressure; I had long since put Anna in the "friends-only" category. Thinking of her in any other way just felt weird at that point.

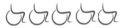

After I asked Anna to the semiformal, I didn't really think about it again. Then, a month or so before, Anna brought it up. It was basically about logistics—when and where, what to wear—but then she bluntly added: "Just because I am single, don't think that means we can hook up after the semiformal."

At first, what she said did not compute. "What did she just say?" "I must have misunderstood." Then she said something else flirtatious, and then something else, and it kept going.

Of course, I played along and flirted back, but it still didn't fully register. I assumed Anna had just been in a good mood that day. But it was the same thing the next time I saw her, and the next time.

She was laying it on so thick that I really had no room to wonder what was going on. It was very clear that she was into me.

My logical side was screaming: "Don't do it! It's a mistake!" "It will ruin the friendship!" "You have already been down this road!" But my less rational side said: "Hell yeah! Let's do this."

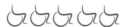

It was the big day; I sported my finest gray suit, took two shots of Three Olives, and I was ready to go. Anna met me in the lobby and we proceeded to the multipurpose room. As we made our way over there, I felt a mixture of excitement and apprehension as to how the night would unfold. The two of us had made several playful allusions that something would happen after the semiformal, but nothing was certain.

The event itself was really nice. It was extravagantly decorated with black paper curtains on the walls, and metallic plastic stars complemented the dark color nicely. There were several metallic spheres hanging from the ceiling, fancy white tablecloths on the tables, and a chocolate fondue fountain. It wasn't the usual tacky, dollar-store decorations typical of University Housing events. This felt classy.

Then, as the event kicked off, the lights dimmed a little, and the music was turned up. The dance floor was quickly filled, and it was great to see all the other residents "dancing" and having a good time. It was a real sight to behold, a harmony of inter-ability dancing and revelry.

I would normally try to take in as much of that positivity as I could, but that night I had other concerns. My focus was on Anna, and nothing else.

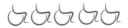

Anna was giving me clear and overt signs the entire night, there was: her not-so-vanilla dancing, the physical affection—hugs, ruffling my hair, grabbing my limp arm and waving it around like I was a puppet, the seductive look she kept giving me. I thought to myself: "Oh yeah! It's definitely on."

Then she gave me an impatient look that said: "What are you waiting for? Make your move already." And I froze like a deer in headlights.

I had exactly what I wanted; I had the all-clear to seal the deal, but I couldn't do it. If it had been any other girl, it would've been no big deal. But the fact that it was Anna— one of my best friends—made me nervous. I was so afraid of screwing it up that I couldn't bring myself to do anything.

Instead of taking her to my room, I just followed Alan to his room. We ended up drinking with Alan and Ron, and their dates.

Pretty soon the night was over and everyone left, leaving me feeling like an absolute coward. I had had exactly what I wanted and did nothing. This had been my second chance, another opportunity, and it was gone. I was so distraught that I dumped my frustrations on the next person I saw: the PA putting me to bed.

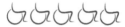

As Tom helped me get to bed, I had quite a tale to tell. And, like any good friend, Tom was excited and supportive.

He started to egg me on, saying I should ask Anna to "come back over." I was terrified of this idea, and began to overanalyze it: "Maybe I'm getting the wrong idea." "Anna gets in everyone's personal space; it's just how she is. I shouldn't read into it." Tom essentially told me to man up, and, from what I had told him, it was definitely not in my imagination.

He snatched the phone off of my desk, and offered to send a text on my behalf. This really freaked me out because I couldn't physically take the phone back. I started pleading with him to stop.

Tom was persistent: "I'll say whatever you want it to say." I was also persistent: "Don't send it!" "I'm just gonna tell her she should come back over, it's not that big of a thing." I was starting to get seriously frustrated: "Come on man, stop!!" Tom was giggling at how much I was flipping out, but still made a good point: "If you don't say something now, with me giving you a little extra push, when are you going to say something?"

He was right, but I was still afraid: "I don't care, I don't want you to send anything." Tom had not budged: "Well,

I'm doing it." He left me no other choice: "If you do it, you are fired!" Tom finally backed down: "Fine. I thought I was helping you out, but if you don't want me to send it, I won't." He proceeded to plug my phone into the charger, and we continued the shift.

After a few minutes, my phone went off. "You didn't?!" Tom said matter-of-factly, "I did. I lied. I did text her. Do you want to see what she responded?" Immediately I could feel my blood pressure pulsating in my brain. I was utterly terrified, knowing I was locked in at this point.

As Tom walked over to get my phone, I was having a bit of a panic attack. I told him I couldn't look at it, and he would have to tell me if it was good or bad. Tom looked at it and grinned: "Here, have a look."

I took the phone in my hand and saw Tom's original message: "I wish you could have stayed. You should come back over." I was slightly relieved: "Hmm. Harmless enough." Then I saw her reply: "I would, but I have to get up early for work tomorrow."

I did a complete emotional 180: "She would. SHE WOULD! Would is good!" Tom agreed: "Dude, 'would,' is awesome!" I was genuinely grateful: "Thanks man. I don't know if I would've been able to do that on my own."

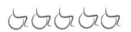

THE DATING GAME

PART FOUR: THE BIRTHDAY

Anna's birthday was the week following the semiformal. The whole Roberts crew planned to meet her at The Summit, but I was feeling a bit uneasy about it: I had not seen her since that night, and didn't know what she was thinking. How would she react? How was I supposed to react? Would it be awkward? I almost didn't even want to go, but figured, given recent developments, I kind of had to.

My plan was to lie low and eventually make my way over to Anna. I opted to just hang out with Alan and Ron in the meantime.

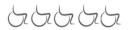

As I was scoping out a good spot to reserve for the army of wheelies on the way,[33] Anna and I made eye contact. And I guess that was all it took, because her face lit up and she ran over to me.

We exchanged some of our usual banter, and then she just straight up asked: "So, what's up with the booty call?" I explained that it had been genuine, and wasn't just the alcohol talking. Then, the two of us both finally admitted

---

33 Buses only allowed two wheelchairs, so we had to travel two at a time.

we liked each other, and had a lengthy discussion about "us."

We addressed the questions: "What will this mean for the future?" "What will happen to our friendship?" "Is it worth it?" "How is it going to work?" And then there was the issue of keeping things under wraps, seeing as "fraternizing" between PAs and residents was frowned upon. It was a long and thorough conversation, and, after an hour or so, we agreed to proceed and see where it goes.

Then, when the talking was through, it was time to consummate the thing. Since we had to keep our arrangement a secret, our mission would have to be a covert one. We came up with a simple, yet effective, cover story: she would "help me use the bathroom." Anna had helped me hundreds of times before, so this wasn't going to raise any eyebrows. The two of us both headed to the bathroom, and, needless to say, the mission was accomplished.

We simply exited the bathroom, and returned to the group—no one was the wiser. Anna continued her social butterfly ways, and I reassumed my position in the wheelie circle.[34]

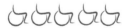

We tried dating for a while, but it fizzled out after a month or two. Over the next few years, we would try again here

---

34 In a crowded place, we would form a large perimeter circle around the group. This was the best use of space.

and there, but it never lasted. I think we just worked better as friends. And honestly, that was fine. Anna was a truly great friend and, I am happy to say, we remain friends to this day.

CHAPTER SEVENTEEN

MISCELLANEA

The following are stories I couldn't find a good place for. I didn't want to shoehorn anything in, so I put all of them in a separate chapter.

ढ़ढ़ढ़ढ़ढ़

MISCELLANEA

PART ONE: BOUNDARIES

In chapter ten, I described how some PAs really trusted me. Tom had confided in me about his relationship, and Anna had shared her concerns about her sister's behavior problems. This trust laid the foundation for some very strong bonds. I became close friends with several PAs.

It was pretty cool to spend so much time with my friends during their shifts, but there was another side to that arrangement: I still technically employed them. And, as such, I had a responsibility to maintain certain boundaries: a balance between being a friend and being an employer.

This intertwining of social roles was tricky. I had to be

careful; if I slipped too far in either direction—too much friend or too much employer—it could get messy.

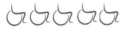

"John Smith" was one of those PAs that everyone liked. He often hung out after he was done working, and even went out drinking with us sometimes. I considered him as much a friend as Alan or Ron.

On top of that, John was also a great PA. He was reliable, efficient, and fun to work with. I had no complaints.

Then, slowly, little things began to happen that I didn't like. John would be the floater, and say things like: "You need something? Okay, give me five minutes," or, "Can it wait until commercial? This is a new episode of *It's Always Sunny* (in Philadelphia)." Other times, I would hear the pager going off after I pressed it, so I knew he was at the desk; he just wasn't coming.

John also worked a bathroom shift, in the middle of the day, on Tuesdays. It normally took about fifteen minutes, a quick shift in between lunch and class. I would simply use the bathroom, and be on my way. But, one day, my class was canceled, and I wanted to use the extra time to organize some papers on my desk.

He complained, "Come on! You never do all of this." Then, John kept saying, "Anything else?" "Anything else?" I felt rushed the entire time, and ended the shift sooner than I wanted to.

I knew it wasn't right, and I wanted to speak up, but I couldn't. It felt weird to say something; John was my friend. I didn't want to confront him or anything; so, I just gave in, and ended the shift.

This was the wrong move; I showed him that complaining worked, and basically encouraged more "bad behavior."

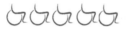

After a year or two, I started to need help being fed, and our brief bathroom shifts became lunch shifts. It was more of the same: John complained, rushed me, and generally had an attitude. He also started to be disrespectful and inappropriate: when I needed something from a spoon or fork, he would often do the "here comes the airplane" thing.

I quickly grew tired of that, and asked John to stop: "Come on man, just feed me normally." But he didn't stop. It became clear he no longer took me seriously as an employer. I had to let him go.

When I fired him, John responded, "I thought we were friends. You don't want me to work for you anymore?" The "friend" comment really tripped me up. I had no good answer, and awkwardly fumbled through the rest of the conversation.

Things between John and I were never the same after that. I had allowed the relationship to stray too far into the friendship direction, and working together became impossible.

I learned the importance of keeping clear boundaries. I needed to be assertive, and speak up when PAs didn't act right.

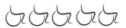

The PA relationship can stray too far in the employee direction as well. This isn't as bad as the first scenario; you can still work with the person, but the whole experience feels mechanical and cold.

I was once in a bind, and needed to quickly fill some shifts. I immediately hired "Mary Jones," one of the first students who replied to my online ad—no interview or anything.

This wasn't ideal, but, at first, it seemed to work out okay. She was showing up on time, and even took a Friday evening shift—which were notoriously hard to fill.

The only issue was: Mary was a bit awkward. It was kind of a pain, but it wasn't anything out of the ordinary. Lots of PAs were uncomfortable at first. As per usual, I expected that to go away after a few weeks.

I waited—and waited—but she never loosened up. I tried my hardest to make small talk, but got nowhere. I would ask, "Do you have any brothers or sisters?" I would get a very succinct, "I have a brother." "Um, is he older or younger?" Again, just a simple, "He's older." I thought to myself, "I am naked, in the shower, and I hardly know you! A little conversation would make this less weird."

Every attempt at conversation was the same: a robotic question-and-answer game. Mary never engaged, not once. I kept telling myself, "She's doing what you're paying her for. Don't fire someone just because they're awkward." I thought maybe if I said it enough, I would start to believe it.

Then, one day, as Mary was lifting me from the bed to my wheelchair, she slipped. We barely made it: my ass was as close to the edge of the seat as possible, and my legs were still on the bed.

I was sitting there, suspended between my bed and wheelchair, and she never said a word. No, "I'm sorry." No, "Are you okay?" Nothing. She just continued, unsuccessfully, trying to drag me the rest of the way. I finally had to say, rather harshly, "I'm already on the chair, just scoot my legs back!!"

I fired Mary shortly after that. I didn't feel so great about it, but I didn't trust her anymore. Maybe if we had developed some sort of rapport, I could have overlooked her screw-up, but we had nothing. I felt no pressure to keep her.

I learned that there is more to being a PA than simply showing up and doing the job. There has to be some personal connection in order for it to work.

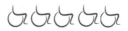

At Roberts, there were several unwritten rules about how to treat an off-duty PA. It was important to know whether a PA was working or not, and to act accordingly.

In one of the first weeks of college, I was late for class, and needed to put something in my bag before I could leave. I was panicking: frantically pressing the floater button every ten seconds.

I eventually went to the floater desk to see if they were there. The desk was empty, but I ran into one of the live-in PAs checking her mail. When I saw her, I felt relieved: "Oh good, I'm glad you're here. I need something really quick." She replied matter-of-factly, "Sorry, I'm not working right now." I was shocked: "I know, but it will only take a second." She again replied frankly, "If I helped you, when I'm off-duty, then I would have to help everyone," and walked away.

Later, I complained to one of the student mentors about how rude she had been, and received no sympathy. He said bluntly, "You can't ask a live-in PA for help if they are off-duty."

I was surprised at how serious everyone was being about this; I hadn't realized how big of a taboo it was to overstep those boundaries.

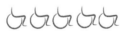

A similar thing happened, a few weeks later, at a football game.

Alan and I were meeting up with Tom for the only night game of the season. Neither of us had a PA—Tom wasn't technically working—but we figured he would still help out if we needed anything.

After getting into the stadium, Tom helped us get snacks from the concession, and the three of us headed to the accessible seating area.

Around the middle of the first quarter, I finished my giant Sprite, and asked Tom to help me use the bathroom. Then Alan asked him to get nachos. Then I asked him to help me put a sweatshirt on. And on and on. We continued asking for stuff, over the course of the game, and he seemed glad to help; I wasn't too worried about overstepping boundaries.

Then, at halftime, I asked him to help me use the bathroom again. Tom agreed, but I guess it was one time too many, because he was not happy: "Why don't you guys have PAs for this? I've been up doing something every two minutes."

I was blindsided; the thought had never crossed my mind that we were asking for too much help. I immediately apologized, and assured Tom we would tone it down.

I decided not to ask for anything else for the rest of the game; if I had to use the bathroom, I would just hold it.

I stayed silent throughout the second quarter and halftime. But then, midway through the third quarter, I had to use the bathroom again. There was no way I could make it until the end of the game, and I wasn't about to ask Tom a third time. So, I left the game to have the floater help me.

It kind of sucked to leave early, but what else was I supposed to do? I didn't want to take advantage of Tom.

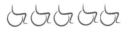

MISCELLANEA

PART TWO: THE CRIP CARD

Recall from chapter ten that the Crip Card was a bit of Roberts slang. It referred to leveraging the overly nice treatment of people with disabilities. The Crip Card was a metaphorical membership card into the Crip Club: an exclusive "club" with benefits ranging from good seats at sporting events, to cutting lines at bars.

My introduction to the Crip Card was going to a football game without a ticket. Getting away with something like that was exciting, but it was only the beginning. As I progressed through college, I found far more uses for the Crip Card than I had ever imagined.

Alan and I were really craving McDonald's late one evening—I wanted some McNuggets, he wanted a McFlurry with M&M's—and we were determined to get it.

It was dark, cold, and McDonald's was almost a mile away from the dorm, but it didn't matter; we were going

We made it past the less-than-stellar sidewalks near the stadium, and through the disgusting viaduct that smelled like pee. The only obstacle left was crossing the four lanes of heavy traffic on Randall Street.

This presented a problem: neither Alan nor I could reach the walk button. Our only option was to wait for a red light, and book it across. That was a scary proposition—there were speeding semi's on Randall Street—but I was on a mission for those McNuggets.

Alan and I safely made it across the street, and arrived at the front door, only to find that McDonald's was closed. I was voice-crackingly furious: "No! It can't be!" Alan tried to suggest Taco Bell, which was down the street, but I didn't want to hear it. I snapped, "No! I want my damn McNuggets!"

Then, suddenly, I noticed a light on inside—signs of life. There were clearly people behind the counter, but the dining area was dark; so, I wasn't sure what was going on. After a minute or two of examining the activity inside, a car exited the drive-through lane.

At that point, I was ready to give up: "I guess only the drive-through is open." But then: "Hmm..." "You know, we are technically driving through, just not in a car."

Alan was concerned they wouldn't let us do it, but I reassured him: "Come on. Do you really think they're going to say anything to people in wheelchairs?" A mischievous grin appeared on Alan's face, as he added, "I'm pretty sure McDonald's accepts the Crip Card. Let's do it!"

We cautiously went up to the speaker. Nothing happened. The two of us waited, and still nothing. Alan was skeptical: "I heard there's a weight limit to activate these things. Our wheelchairs probably aren't heavy enough." "Yeah, maybe you—" I was cut off: "Welcome to McDonald's, can I take your order?"

As I started placing my order, I could feel the bright glare of headlights from behind. I thought to myself, "I guess we're part of the line if other cars are waiting behind us." As Alan placed his order, I had to see the car for myself; I turned around, and, sure enough, there was a big white pickup truck right behind us.

We both pulled up to the counter, giggling at our own shenanigans, and the guy at the window looked very surprised to see us. But then he gave Alan our food without even a hint of a smile. He must not have appreciated the humor of the situation.

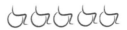

The Crip Card seemingly had no limits. We were constantly pushing the envelope, seeing what we could get away with.

After a particularly wild night out, we—Ron, Tom, and I—were hungry. The three of us headed to the student union, to get something from the late-night convenience-store-esque shop adjacent to the cafeteria. But sadly, it turned out to be closed; we would have to order takeout instead.

The only thing open in the union was the study lounge. So, we settled down in there, and the peaceful calm of the lounge was interrupted as we argued over which restaurant to call.

The three of us decided on pizza, and then looked up the number. Tom held the phone to my ear, and, for some reason—most likely the several drinks I had had that evening—I did my best impression of Tom while I ordered. I impersonated his Eastern European accent, while also exaggerating his interesting manner of speaking: "Helloo kind sir, I vould like to order your finest peachsa pie, and your most presteegious chicken streeps." Ron immediately started belting out in laughter, as Tom defended himself: "Hey! Fuck you! I don't sound like that!"

Then I received the bad news: the food wouldn't be there for at least forty-five minutes. We were not happy—being drunk and hangry is a bad combination. "Really? How hard is it to deliver pizzas?!" "What exactly is taking so long?! You cook the fucking thing, and put it in a box! It should take five minutes at the most!"

After we ranted for a while, it dawned on the three of us how loud we were being, in what was basically a library. We looked around and received a few dirty looks, with many more faces looking down to avoid eye contact. "I can't believe no one said anything." "Yeah! No one even shh-ed us."

Ron commented jokingly, "If anyone else had been this loud, they would've gotten their asses kicked. But, because we are in wheelchairs, no one said anything. That's discrimination!" I added with a grin, "I am tired of this! I deserve to have my ass kicked just like anybody else."

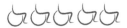

We all had a good laugh, but then Tom took things up a notch: "Let's see how far we can take this. See how far the Crip Card can go."

Ron and I instantly agreed. The only question was: how to conduct this important experiment?

The choice was obvious: the penis game. It's a simple game: the players take turns shouting the dirty word, progressively getting louder and louder, until someone refuses to continue. The penis game is a test to see how rude and obnoxious you are willing to be, and it usually ends pretty quick; but this time, there was no telling how long it would last

The game went around many times, with no sign of slowing down—and still not a peep from any of the studiers. Tom was getting frustrated: "This is ridiculous! I guess we will have to do something drastic." He jumped on the back of Ron's wheelchair, and they proceeded to ride around the room, Tom's booming voice reverberating off the walls: "Peeeniss! PEENNISS!!" Ron was moving in between rows of tables, forcing frantic students to move their bags out of the way, and I just stared in disbelief.

They returned from their penis-shouting rampage, and looked very proud of themselves. But I was not as impressed. I whispered, "Have you guys lost your minds?" and motioned for them to look at the row of tables they had just terrorized. Some of the studiers seriously looked like they were about to kill us. Ron mumbled, "We should probably leave..."

We decided to forgo the pizza, and get the hell out of there. The three of us went hungry, but, at least, the experiment had been a success: we discovered the Crip Card indeed has limits.

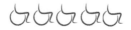

MISCELLANEA

PART THREE: ROLLING WITH THE PUNCHES

Murphy's Law is an everyday part of having a disability. There will inevitably be times when things can and will go wrong. Ordinary situations will be unnecessarily difficult, and plans will fall apart. It's an unfortunate fact of life. But, it's important to not let the obstacles get you down.

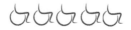

It was an older resident's last a cappella concert before he graduated, and a large group of Roberts wheelies were going.

When we arrived at the theater, a customer service person came to inform Anna[35] there wouldn't be enough accessible seating. Due to the high number of wheelies attending, the accessible seats could not fit all of us.

We were disappointed, and started discussing who would be okay with missing the show. But Anna refused to accept this. She was on a mission to make sure we all saw the concert.

Anna took complete command of the situation. She immediately directed Phil, Ron, and a few others to take the remaining accessible seats. Then she told the rest of us—Alan, myself, and two freshmen—to follow her.

We arrived at the main door to the auditorium, and were all a bit confused because it had stairs. But Anna didn't skip a beat. She immediately got to work: carrying each of us, one at a time, into regular seats. And I mean she literally carried us: groom-holding-the-bride style, down the sloping stairs of the theater aisle, all while taking care not to bump our heads or dangling legs.

I was thoroughly impressed with her herculean effort, and developed a newfound respect for Anna after this: she cared that much about including everybody.

---

35 Whenever there's a group of wheelies, the able-bodied person is assumed to be in charge.

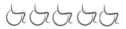

We stayed for the entire show, and got to see the older resident perform his last concert. The only obstacle left was whether Anna could get us all back to our wheelchairs. This would be even more difficult than before, seeing as now she had to carry us up the stairs. But, somehow, she managed.

I was the last one to be transported back to my wheelchair, and, of course, something went wrong during my turn. I am not sure what happened—maybe she was exhausted from the previous lifts, or she had a bad grip—but my pants fell down while she was carrying me. My tighty-whities were visible to the entire crowd.

I began yelling, "Quick! Get me back to my chair, my pants fell down!" Anna couldn't control her laughter, and almost dropped me. And, after I was placed back in my chair, Anna couldn't even help me with my pants because she was struggling not to keel over.

After what seemed like an eternity, I was finally made decent, and the five of us headed home.

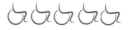

The concert had been an absolute train wreck. I could have easily gotten upset about everything that happened—the lack of accessible seating, needing to be carried to and from my seat, my pants falling down—but I didn't. I was able to laugh it off, because it wasn't anything out of the ordinary.

Disasters are commonplace when you have a severe disability; you have to roll with the punches, and not let it bother you.

CHAPTER EIGHTEEN

ASPIRATIONS v. LIMITATIONS

PART ONE: A MAJOR PAIN

Starting college as a math major wasn't the wisest decision. My guidance counselor had warned me college math was intense, and suggested I take a few classes before declaring, but I didn't listen. I was young, dumb, and over-confident; I wanted to dive right in.

I thought I would breeze through math, like I always had. Then classes started, and I was put in my place.

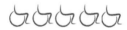

I immediately struggled. The workload was unbelievable; we covered more, in the first few weeks, than they had in an entire semester of high school math.

My life became an endless stream of homework, and, from the very beginning, it kicked my ass. I just couldn't handle the physical demands of studying so much.

It was a workout for me. My arm would get sore after writing for so long. And, when I sat and studied for several hours, that was hours of sitting in the exact same position; I couldn't lean side-to-side to stretch out, or squirm to find a more comfortable position.

Then, as classes progressed, it only got worse. When the material got harder, I had to work harder, which put more of a strain on me. And when the material got even harder, I had to work even harder, which put an even bigger strain on me. And on and on.

It continued like this, for two years, until I was eventually working so hard it was ridiculous.

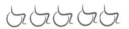

Every day, after dinner, I sat and did homework until about midnight. It was a nonstop, miserable slog, and I would only take a break if I got too stiff and uncomfortable to concentrate.

When my nightly grind wasn't enough, I would study during the day too, skipping my other classes if necessary. Sometimes, I would be at my desk from the moment I got up until the moment I went to bed; on more than one occasion, I even got skin breakdown from sitting so long— literal math-related injuries.

It was rough, but I had no choice. If I slowed down, even for a day or two, I would never catch up.

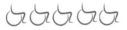

All the physical punishment took its toll. I started getting sick every few weeks. And, each time, I would have to rush to the doctor—for me, any illness is an emergency.[36]

I was sick so often it became routine. I had the process down to a science: the doctor would prescribe me an antibiotic, I would take it easy for three or four days, and then study, twice as hard, to catch up.

I was barely keeping my health under control, and, at that point, I seriously questioned what I was doing. It was clear how futile my efforts were; I was fighting a losing battle. And, deep down, I knew I should quit, but I couldn't bring myself to do it.

I had already taken so many of the core classes; I was almost halfway done with the major, I didn't want to just give it up.

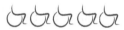

After a particularly nasty cold, I fell really far behind, and had no idea how I was going to catch up.

Then, I had a brilliant idea. One of my PAs had a college blog, and I remembered seeing a post called: *The Ultimate Guide to Pulling an All-Nighter*. It was all spelled out for me; I just had to follow the instructions.

It was the night before my Calculus II midterm, and I was ready: I was rested, there was an energy drink in the fridge, and I had a plan for tackling the material.

I asked my night PA to set up my books to study, and she

---

36 People with Duchenne are at high risk for pneumonia.

was a bit confused. I told her I was pulling an all-nighter, and she looked at me like I was crazy. I knew staying up all night probably wasn't the wisest decision for someone like me, but it was the only option if I wanted to pass Calc II.

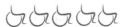

Once I got to work, the hours seemed to fly by, and, around three, I really hit my stride. I was breezing through my notes, and understanding everything: Taylor series, infinite sums, conic sections—I had them all down.

Then, at six, I hit a wall. I was starving, and couldn't focus at all. My studying would have to be put on hold until I ate something. I closed the books, and headed to the only place on campus that was open: a 24-hour IHOP.

After practically inhaling some strawberry crepes, I returned to my room, and reviewed everything one last time.

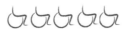

I arrived at the disability testing center,[37] promptly at nine, and got set up in one of the private cubicles. I started the exam, and felt great; I had energy, and was thinking clearly. On top of that, I was pretty proud of myself: "I actually pulled an all-nighter! The gamble paid off!"

---

37 A separate location where students with disabilities can take their exams with accommodations.

I easily made it through the first few problems, but then it all fell apart; I suddenly felt like I was dying: trouble breathing, dripping with sweat, heart pounding.

I had been through similar bouts of fatigue in the past, but this was different. This felt like the end; I had pushed my already vulnerable body to its limit, and now it was finally saying, "no more."

I knew it was over, and decided, right then and there, to call it quits: "I put up a good fight, but I guess math is too much for me." I turned in a half-finished exam, and went home.

I immediately got in bed, and passed out until dinner. When I woke up, I dropped the class, and then switched majors shortly after.

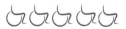

ASPIRATIONS v. LIMITATIONS

PART TWO: NOT WORTH IT

My struggle with math was, by no means, the first time I had refused to accept my limitations. I outright ignored them more times than I can count.

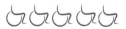

In the early days, I was entranced by the college mythology: partying to excess, staying up absurdly late, and generally being a slob. There was just something so deliciously immature about doing idiotic things. I reveled in the senseless debauchery of it all, and never missed an opportunity to indulge.

It was the last week of the school year, and I wanted to end with a bang. I talked to Tom, who was also finished with classes early, and he invited me to come drink with him and his roommates. I knew how hard those guys went, and jumped at the chance to join them.

When I arrived, they were playing a drinking game involving Mario Kart for the N64. The game was simple: whoever came in last place had to take a shot. I laughed when Tom explained it, because I honestly thought he was joking: "Doesn't a race take only like three or four minutes?" "Yeah." "But that would mean someone is taking a shot every three or four minutes." "Yeah, so? The point of the game is to get shit-faced."

I knew I shouldn't; someone with Duchenne has no business drinking that much. But, on the other hand, I did want them to think I was cool, so I agreed to play.

It went about as well as you'd expect: after an hour or so, I was in no shape to continue playing, and Tom had to help me home.

When I woke up the next morning, I was hurting; I had never felt so sick in my entire life. I couldn't get out of bed. I canceled my morning PA, and only had my afternoon PA give me a few sips of Gatorade, before sending her on her way.

My sister Liz—who was also a student at GMU—stopped by, and was not happy to find me still in bed at four in the afternoon. She really let me have it: "Why would you think drinking that much was a good idea? Was it worth it? Was it worth wasting your entire day?!"

She was absolutely right. It was not worth it to drink that much. I idolized the whole college lifestyle, idolized the alcohol-fueled shenanigans, but my body obviously couldn't handle it.

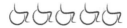

My limits weren't always physical, i.e., how much my body could handle. Sometimes they were environmental.

I had been talking to a girl I liked—let's call her Ashley—and things were going really well. She eventually invited me to a party at her apartment; I was super excited, and couldn't wait to go. But then, the day before, I learned it was on the second floor, and there was no elevator.

I told her I couldn't go, but she assured me one of her male friends could carry me up the stairs. I was a bit skeptical: "I don't know if I like the idea of a complete stranger lifting me. And what if he is already drunk when I get there?" "My friend Mike is not like that. He's really responsible."

It was a terrible idea. There were a thousand things

that could go wrong. But, on the other hand, I really liked Ashley, and thought the party was a good chance to move things along; so, I did it anyway.

I thought to myself, "I'm not giving this up just because she happens to live on the second floor. I'm not going to let some stairs get in my way; a few pieces of wood and some nails are not enough to stop me!"

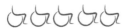

Ashley and "responsible" Mike were waiting for me when I arrived at the base of the stairs. They both looked to me, assuming I knew exactly what to do. I had no idea, but tried to act like I did; I quickly scoped things out, and came up with a plan.

I told Ashley how to disengage my wheelchair, and had her move it under the stairs—I figured that was better than leaving it out in the open. Then I game-planned the lift with Mike, and he proceeded to carry me up the stairs, and into the apartment, with relative ease.

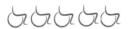

The party couldn't have gone any better: Ashley and I were basically together the whole time. We talked, we laughed, we flirted, we shared drink after drink. Everything was going great, until it was time to go.

As I was getting ready to leave, "responsible" Mike

was nowhere to be found. Ashley tried calling him, but he didn't answer. And, at that point, I started to get concerned because Mike was my only option; all the other guys at the party were in no shape to carry me.

Out of desperation, Ashley offered to carry me, and I thought it was a ridiculous idea: "You can't be serious." She flexed her arms and confidently said, "Look at these! I can handle it!"

I wasn't exactly convinced by the demonstration. How strong could she be at 5'4" 115-ish lbs? I didn't like the idea at all, but what choice did I have? It was either her or one of her sloppy-drunk friends.

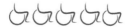

Ashley picked me up, and, after a few steps, I could feel her arms shaking—a sign of struggle. I knew she was nervous, so I stayed calm, but on the inside I was terrified.

We started down the stairs; and, with each step, I felt her grip loosening. I seriously thought I was going over the railing; I was going to plummet head-first into the concrete below.

I closed my eyes and braced for impact, but, at the last minute, Ashley was able to grab a handful of shirt. My life now depended on the tensile strength of my tacky pinstriped button-up.

The shirt miraculously held together, and we made it down the last few stairs. She placed me in my wheelchair, and let out an exaggerated "Pheww!" trying to relieve some of the tension. I laughed nervously, knowing full-well how close I came to being dropped.

After that little incident, I vowed to never be carried up the stairs like that again. It wasn't worth it. When Ashley invited me to a semi-formal, in a second-story room of The Rogue Ales, a few weeks later, I had to turn her down.

She tried to convince me it wouldn't be a repeat of the last time: "I could have a few of the guys carry you together. Probably chair-and-all," but it honestly sounded *more* dangerous.

Being carried up the stairs is one thing, but being carried up the stairs, while also strapped to a three-hundred-pound wheelchair, is another. I was absolutely not doing that.

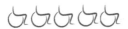

This pattern continued for most of my adult life. I would encounter some new limitation, refuse to accept it, suffer the consequences, and ultimately be forced to accept it anyway.

Whether the impairment was physical—being unable to sit and study for hours—or environmental—a building with no elevator—I always refused to back down. Giving in would mean accepting my limitations; I would be admitting I couldn't do what I wanted. And what twenty-year-old kid wants to admit that?

CHAPTER NINETEEN

A BIG MOVE

Since its inception, the Roberts program had always been housed in a small, unimpressive facility, barely equipped to handle residents with disabilities. But that was about to change: Roberts was getting a much-needed upgrade.

There had been a new dorm—Parikh Hall—under construction since I arrived in 2008, and the program was finally moving there in the fall of 2010.

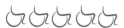

We were given a tour in spring 2010, and it was something to behold; Parikh Hall was state-of-the-art.

The doors were all keyless, activated by either hitting a button, or holding your student ID card up to a scanner. And the elevators had something I had never seen before: oversized buttons, at knee-height, which could be pressed by tapping into them with your wheelchair.

What's more, every room had a Hoyer lift mounted to the ceiling, as well as a hospital bed. And it wasn't just any hospital bed, some old rickety eyesore; this was more of a hospital bed disguised as a regular bed—nice headboard, no obnoxious rails.

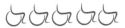

Then the tour took us upstairs, and I was confused because Roberts was only on the first floor of Parikh. I thought all the other floors were mainstream housing, but, to my surprise, we were shown five more accessible rooms on the second floor. These were the so-called "transition rooms."

As Sharon—the program admin—later explained in our monthly meeting: "You remember that one of the main goals of the program is to teach independent living skills?" "Yeah." "And the hope is students, who are able, will eventually move out of the program and find mainstream housing." "Yeah, of course. I'd like to move out eventually." "Well, the transition rooms are sort of a middle ground between Roberts and mainstream housing: it's still a fully accessible room, but there's no floater or guidance from the staff. They are a stepping stone between being fully supported, and being on your own."

After hearing her pitch for the transition rooms, Sharon asked if I thought I was ready to move out. I had been planning on moving out a year or two down the line, but these transition rooms seemed like a game-changer. I was so infatuated with the idea of transitioning to mainstream housing, of moving out a year or two sooner, that I immediately signed up.

The next week I signed a new housing contract, and we began collaborating on a plan for the move, meeting periodically during the spring semester.

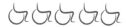

I was super excited telling my parents about my plans—leaving Roberts, beginning my journey toward independent living—but they didn't share my enthusiasm.

They were very aware of all the details I wasn't seeing. For starters, I would have to find my own PA staff; I could no longer hire from the list of PAs compiled by Roberts. My PAs would also be paid through the state instead of the university, which would involve a lot more red tape. And, as they both pointed out, those were just the issues they could think of; there would almost certainly be more.

My dad tried to reason with me: "This system with the transition rooms is brand-new. All the kinks will have to be worked out. Let someone else be the guinea pig." But I didn't want to hear it; I just didn't want to believe it couldn't work. So, I kept on reassuring him: "Everything will be fine. Everything will be fine. I'll figure it out as I go."

They tried, for months, to talk me out of it, but I refused to budge. When it was clear I wasn't going to change my mind, my parents had no choice but to let me find out for myself.

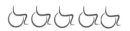

Sharon and I signed the necessary paperwork, and it was official: I had moved out of Roberts.

CHAPTER TWENTY

A BIG MISTAKE

PART ONE: A BAD OMEN

It was a long and stressful day of moving in to my new room, but, overall, everything went smoothly: we found a good arrangement for all the new furniture, my student ID was given access to the keyless entry system, and my PAs were approved to enter the building.

After several hours, everything was unpacked, and my parents left. I was officially on my own—again.

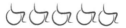

I was feeling pretty good about the new situation. Though, there was still one last hurdle to cross before I could feel completely confident: the first night.

There was no floater, so I came up with my own system. I had arranged for a different PA to stay, in my room, each night. They would sleep on an air mattress, and I would wake them up when I needed something.

It was a pretty simple system; there wasn't much that could go wrong, but I still wanted one night under my belt—just to know it worked.

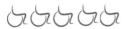

Unfortunately, it didn't go too well. Tom had accidentally double-booked himself; he was already at his other job when I called him, and couldn't leave.

I suddenly had no help during the night, and started freaking out. The RA saw how stressed I was, and came over to ask what was wrong. I explained my situation, and—bless her heart—she offered to fill in.

The RA was happy to help, until I told her she would have to sleep in my room. Then she started backtracking, and getting all wishy-washy about it: "Actually, that might not be a good idea." "I don't know if I feel comfortable with that." "Maybe we can find a male RA to help you instead."

Fearing my only option was slipping away, I quickly offered a compromise: she would sleep in her room, and I would call her on the phone. I wasn't exactly comfortable with this arrangement—I could drop my phone, or she could not wake up—but I had no other choice.

Then, because fate is a sadistic bastard, my cell phone died on me; it literally stopped working when I was about to get in bed.

I was completely bewildered: "Is this really happening?! I can't believe everything is going wrong on the first fucking day!" The anxiety was building; I was on the verge of a panic attack, when the RA, again, came to the rescue. She put her RA crisis-training to good use, and helped me calm down.

Once I was thinking clearly, I easily found a solution: I borrowed a phone for the night, and made an appointment, the next day, at the AT&T store.

The situation was resolved, and everything turned out okay, but I was still shaken up. If something, as foolproof as my night system, could fail, then nothing was safe.

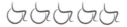

As I laid in bed, with a death-grip on my borrowed phone, I could hear my dad's voice in my head: "Why didn't you listen to me? You just had to move out, didn't you?" I sighed. Yet again, I had to admit my parents were right all along: it *was* impossible to plan for everything, and there *would* be problems I couldn't foresee.

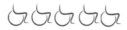

A BIG MISTAKE

PART TWO: OH FLOATER, WHERE ART THOU?

During the first week, I was hit with a hard reality check. All the issues I had ignored, when planning the move, came back to haunt me: having no floater was harder than expected; the PAs—who I had been entirely responsible for finding and training—were less than stellar; and several PA paychecks were delayed as I learned the new payroll system.

All of these problems were difficult to manage, but having no floater was particularly awful. I no longer had access to around-the-clock assistance; I could only get help during my PA shifts—a small window of just three or four hours per day.

I really had to be sure I remembered everything I needed. If I forgot something, during a shift, I was out of luck.

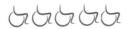

Going to the bathroom became my greatest struggle. I tried to keep it under control, but there's a limit to how much you can regulate your bodily functions— "pee math" could only do so much; unscheduled needs were inevitable.

At first, I assumed I was just adjusting to a new routine: a few random pees while I trained my body to go at specific times; I thought everything would stabilize after a few days, but it only got worse. Pretty soon, I had spontaneous urges popping up every day—sometimes twice a day.

It was horrible, like a recurring nightmare that always followed the same script. First, came the waiting game: I had to hold it—often for hours—until my next PA arrived. As I sat perfectly still, trying to stay calm, I would find myself glancing at the clock, every five minutes, hoping it had magically skipped ahead. And then, when the urge got really bad, I would start pacing back and forth to take my mind off of it.

Next, came the frantic rush to the bathroom. When my PA showed up, I would "calmly inform" them of the urgent situation, and "gently encourage" them to get everything ready—legs moved into position, pants untied, urinal in place—as fast as possible. The subsequent flurry of lifting, leaning, and scooting, would be so quick and efficient it would make a NASCAR pit crew jealous.

And finally, the whole ordeal would end with a feeling of indescribable, cathartic relief.

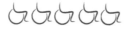

I started to live my life like an addict, day-to-day and hour-to-hour, wondering when I would get my next bathroom fix. It was an exhausting way to live, and I eventually lost the will to fight it.

One day, in mid-September, I was sitting in the testing center taking an exam. I was also struggling to hold it, and had no idea how I was going to make it through the exam, let alone the lengthy wait that would follow—the exam ended at one, and my next PA wasn't coming until four.

I tried my best to fight through it, but the pain was hard to ignore; it became so intense I had to stop working on the exam, and lean back in my wheelchair.

I sat there, contemplating the next few hours of suffering, and started to panic: "I can't focus! I'm going to fail this exam! Making it through the exam isn't even the end of this!..."

Then, it happened. Something snapped in me, and I didn't care anymore. I had been through the same bathroom-emergency bullshit, every day for weeks, and I was done. It wasn't worth the pain anymore; I started going right there in my testing cubicle.

When it was over, I sat in shameful silence for a good ten minutes. I couldn't believe what I had just done: "Why? Why did I do that? I willingly pissed my pants. What's wrong with me?!"

ᘒᘒᘒᘒᘒ

I didn't even turn in the exam. I rushed back to my room, locked the door, and didn't leave until my next PA arrived.

Anna showed up a few hours later, and I asked her to help me change clothes. She helped me clean up, while also lecturing me about getting my shit together: "Come on, what are you doing to yourself? You can't keep doing this! If you do, you will get a rash. Or an infection..."

Anna was right: I needed to figure things out. I couldn't go around pissing myself like that. But what was I supposed to do? My body was on its own schedule; I couldn't control when I had to go.

My solution: circumvent the problem entirely, and stop

drinking "unnecessary" fluids. I figured, if I drank less fluids, I would use the bathroom less. It wasn't the healthiest thing to do, but it was the best I could come up with.

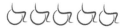

Another problem, with having no floater, was exhaustion. In the past, I would nap whenever I got worn down. But now, I was only able to nap during PA shifts—which wasn't enough; after I was done with everything else, I was only left with fifteen or twenty minutes to lie down.

This lack of rest had a dramatic effect on me: I was all over the place emotionally, it was harder to focus in class, and conversations seemed like they were going a mile a minute—sometimes I could barely follow them. I also felt physically weaker; normally easy things became difficult for me, like: getting my phone out of my pocket, or flipping through a textbook.

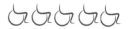

One Saturday morning, I didn't have the energy to get out of bed. I had stayed up late, and barely slept; there was no way I would be able to function without more sleep, so I had my PA leave me in bed.

I passed out for several hours, and woke up completely refreshed. I was feeling amazing, until I remembered I had gone to sleep with no plan for getting back up. I had no way to get out of bed: "Shit! What do I do?" My first thought was to text Tom. I figured he would be around, since he was now a live-in PA, and lived right downstairs.

Tom didn't answer, and I was stuck. I ended up having to wait, to get out of bed, until my next PA came—two hours later.

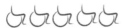

It was scary waking up in discomfort, with no way to get out of bed or even reposition myself, and I never wanted to be in that situation again.

I swore to never again nap without a plan, and made a genuine effort to follow through. I tried my best to deal with the tiredness, to live with the mental fog and "heavy-eyelid" feeling, but I couldn't do it; it seemed I had underestimated my exhaustion. Within days, I had that same debilitating lack of energy, and ended up doing it again: napping without an "exit strategy."

As the semester went on, I would continue to lie down without a plan; it was dangerous, and I knew it, but I needed sleep to function.

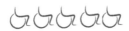

A BIG MISTAKE

PART THREE: THE LEVEE BREAKS

I was under constant stress living outside of Roberts. My stomach was always in knots, and it became very sensitive. I had to start avoiding spicy food, and limiting my drinking—a big sacrifice for a college student.

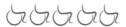

One night, Alan invited me to go to the bars with him, and I refused: "It's probably not the best idea. My stomach has been bothering me lately." He pleaded, "Come on man! Lisa wants me to meet her friends. I can't handle that on my own." "Alright fine. I'll go. But I'm not drinking."

We arrived at Old Town, and Alan immediately ordered kamikaze shots for everyone. I wasn't going to have any, but then Lisa's very cute friend offered to help me take one, and my self-control crumbled.

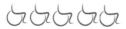

I thought one little shot wouldn't be a big deal, but that kamikaze did not sit well. As soon as I took it, my stomach started bubbling and rumbling in a way it never had before.

I started to feel extremely sick to my stomach. But I wasn't about to abandon my wingman duties; Alan needed me, so I stayed and powered through it.

My stomach pain steadily increased all night, until Alan eventually noticed I was struggling: "Dude, are you feeling okay? You don't look so good." "Not at all. I need to go home."

I left and immediately went to bed,[38] but wasn't able to sleep. I was waking up every twenty minutes.

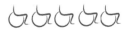

I felt even worse in the morning; it was no longer just my stomach: I was short-of-breath, and my heart rate was noticeably fast. Was I coming down with something?

I stayed in bed after my PA left, and asked my sister to come over and give me a breathing treatment—it always helped whenever I had a cold.

Then, as I waited for her, I was struck with really bad nausea. I thought to myself, "Oh shit! Am I going to throw u—?" I puked before I could finish the thought.

I inspected the stomach contents that were now all over my pillow, and was a bit confused: "Red?! I didn't drink anything red last night." I immediately started trying to remember everything I ate the day before; then, as I was ridding myself of the last few bits of residual vomit, I noticed a familiar flavor. It was something I had tasted before, but couldn't identify.

I sloshed the saliva around in my mouth for a second,

---

38 My night PA would arrive at 10, and wait in my room, until I was ready for bed. This included waiting for me to get back from the bars.

and it suddenly hit me like a cold slap in the face: it was blood. I had thrown up blood.

My first reaction was to panic: "This is bad. This is really bad. People don't just throw up blood for no reason. Something is seriously wrong! What is it?!" Then I calmed down, as my brain switched to survival mode; all emotion seemed to shut off, and I became solely focused on the problem at hand. The only thing I could think about was what I had to do next.

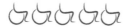

My sister came in, and I asked her to come over to me; I said it calmly so she wouldn't panic—though there wasn't really anything I could do to prevent that. Her face said it all: a look of utter terror, of overwhelming fear. I can still see Liz's face as clearly as you see the words on this page; it was gut-wrenching, and I hope to never see another person make that face again.

Liz frantically grabbed at a washcloth to clean me up: the blood had dripped down, onto the side of my face, and into my hair a little. When I was no longer a bloody mess, my sister looked at me, in tears, and said, "David, I'm scared. What should I do?" I didn't know, but suggested we find someone who did.

I told Liz to run downstairs to Roberts, and tell someone what happened; minutes later, Sharon entered my room, followed by my sister. It made us both feel a little better to have her take charge of the situation.

Listening to Sharon call 911 was sobering. It really sunk in how serious the situation was: "We have a twenty-year-old male, who vomited blood, and needs immediate medical attention…"

The paramedics quickly arrived, and began discussing the best way to get me on the stretcher. During their little game-planning session, Liz squeezed in between them, scooped me up, and tossed me onto the stretcher. They went silent with embarrassment, and I let out a slight smirk.

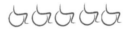

Before I knew it, Liz and I were in the emergency room. I was admitted right away. The paramedics brought me to an empty room, and transferred me onto the bed—without hesitation this time.

The medics left, and a small army of scrub-clad twenty-somethings came in after them. It was chaos. One girl was doing my vitals. Another was helping me get into a gown. The nurse introduced himself, and barraged me with questions: "When did you vomit last?" "What did the blood look like?" "Have you had stomach issues in the past?"

My head was spinning from all the commotion. I was doing my best to pay attention to everybody, when, suddenly, in the middle of answering a question, I threw up again. It was blood—again.

The nurse frantically called to someone in the hallway: "It's coffee grounds!"[39] A doctor immediately entered. He checked for blood in the colon, and the test came out positive. This meant there was: "definitely a G-I bleed."

Another doctor entered, talking about advanced directives and living wills, and I dismissed him: "I don't need that. People only need that if they're gonna die." The two doctors looked at each other, and didn't acknowledge what I said. "What is it? What—" "Oh…mmm."

Before I had time to worry about dying, yet another doctor entered the room talking about "repairing the bleed surgically." It was apparently my best option, so I agreed, and was brought directly to the operating room.

I literally signed a waiver while lying on the operating table. As soon as my hand let go of the pen, they were putting the mask over my face to put me to sleep.

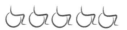

I woke up in a daze, still heavily sedated and disoriented. "What's going on?" "Where am I?" I looked around and saw my whole family was sitting next to me. "Why are my parents here?"

Then the doctor entered the room, and it started coming back to me: the kamikaze, the blood, the emergency room. "Oh shit! I had a surgery." "I must be in the recovery room."

The doctor was talking to my parents, and, as the drugs

---

39 Digested blood is dark and chunky like coffee grounds.

wore off, her muffled voice slowly turned into words. She was explaining what happened: the bleed was caused by a peptic ulcer that ruptured. From what I could gather, it was massive—as far as ulcers go—and I was lucky to be alive.

Then, she discussed all of the potential causes. My mom asked, "Could it have been something he ate?" "No. It is actually a common misconception that food causes ulcers." "He also tested negative for H. pylori—the bacteria that causes ulcers." "The only other thing it could be is stress."

I already knew it was stress: "I don't need a doctor to tell me that!" Over the previous eight weeks, I had been more stressed than I had in my entire life: scrambling to find a way to use the bathroom every day, scrambling to find ways to take naps, and, all the while, trying to keep up with school.

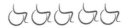

I spent a few days in the ICU, and then headed home. I was given some antibiotics and a recommendation to reduce my stress. But I wasn't sure how I would do that—considering I still had to go back to school; I was, in fact, terrified of returning to school.

CHAPTER TWENTY-ONE

LICKING MY WOUNDS

PART ONE: MOVING BACK

I stayed home, for a week, to recover. I was supposed to rest, but all I could do was worry about going back to school: "How am I going to get through this?! I almost died the first time!"

The situation seemed hopeless. Nothing had changed; there was no reason to believe the rest of the semester would be any different.

ᘒᘒᘒᘒᘒ

One night, I suddenly woke up, gasping for air. I shrieked for my mom, and she came running in.

I told her, "I can't breathe! I think I'm having a heart attack!" She saw nothing was seriously wrong, and replied gently: "No sweetie, I think you are having a panic attack."

My mom waited until I calmed down, then said, "You're worried about going back to school, aren't you?" I was so upset I didn't even try to hold back; I exclaimed, "YESSS!" and burst into tears: "I can't go back! I just can't! There's no way!"

Living outside of Roberts was too much to handle, and

I refused to go back: "I will drop out before I live through that again!" My mom stayed level-headed: "Before you do anything you'll regret, why don't you ask Sharon if you can move back?" It was a nice idea, but I knew it was futile: "That won't happen! There are never empty rooms at Roberts! There is a waiting list just to get a spot!"

My freaking out didn't even faze her; she again replied calmly, "It wouldn't hurt to ask." I still wasn't convinced: "Alright, I'll ask. But I'm telling you, it won't do any good."

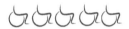

The next morning, I emailed Sharon, asking if I could move back. And, to my surprise, it worked. As luck would have it, a live-in PA had opted out of their contract, and there was an empty room available. In other words: I could move back to Roberts!

I was overjoyed thinking about all of the "luxuries" I would have back: I wouldn't have to remember everything during my shifts; I wouldn't have to worry whether or not I would have help at night; and, hell, I would even be able to go to the bathroom as I pleased—the way the good Lord intended.

For several minutes, I was on cloud nine. Then, I remembered I had to actually accept the offer to make it official. I promptly responded and, after another week of winter break, I was a Roberts resident again.

ㅂㅂㅂㅂㅂ

LICKING MY WOUNDS

PART TWO: AN IMPORTANT MEETING

The whole experience of moving out had been traumatic for me, and I think Sharon recognized that, because she had been asking to meet with me since I got back.

I appreciated the gesture, but I wasn't exactly thrilled to meet with her; the idea of sharing my feelings, with an admin, sounded about as fun as talking to my parents about sex. But, forget the fact she was an administrator; I didn't want to talk to anyone about the move. I intended to keep that embarrassing dumpster fire in the past—where it belonged.

I ignored Sharon's emails, as long as I could, but it became clear she wasn't going to stop asking; I eventually responded, and begrudgingly set up a meeting.

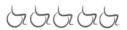

I entered very defensive; I wasn't going to say any more than I needed to. Sharon started off with: "I know this year has been difficult—with the move, and your recent hospitalization. How are you doing?" I quickly said, "Good." "Are you sure? You've been through a lot. It would be perfectly normal to feel a bit shaken." I doubled down: "No, really. I'm fine."

Then, she said something that completely caught me off guard: "Just because you came back, after moving out, doesn't mean you failed." At this, I finally let my guard down: "I know. It just sucks that I couldn't do it. Maybe if I had done something different—" She interrupted, "Don't get down on yourself. You tried your best. If anything, consider it a learning experience. Now you know your limits."

The meeting turned out to be a great help, and I appreciated that Sharon had no agenda—she just wanted to see how I was doing. I wasn't drilled with questions, and nothing significant was asked of me.

The only thing she suggested I do was: "Take some time to reflect on what happened, and consider how to avoid being overwhelmed like that in the future."

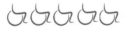

LICKING MY WOUNDS

PART THREE: REEVALUATING SOME THINGS

I took Sharon's advice to heart, and seriously reflected on what happened, on what led to such a catastrophic result.

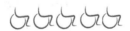

I thought about it long and hard, asking myself the tough questions: "Why did I ignore the warnings from my parents?" "Why did I ignore my own reservations?" "Why was I so adamant about doing something that, deep down, I knew wasn't going to work?" The answer to all of these questions, it turned out, was the same: independent living.

For those of you who may be unfamiliar with independent living, and how big of a deal it is in the disability community, I will give some (brief and extremely oversimplified) background information...

Historically, in the US, the paradigm for how to care for, treat (medically), and generally "deal with" people with disabilities were centered around institutionalization. In short, institutionalization is the practice of putting people with disabilities in nursing homes—often against their will.

Understandably, some people were not the biggest fans of institutionalization, and there was a big push to change things. I'm going to skip over a couple of important events, e.g., social movements and pieces of legislation, but the key takeaway is: institutionalization eventually started to fall out of favor.

The paradigm that replaced it is: "independent living." This is the practice of giving people with disabilities the freedom to live where they want; it can be as simple as providing a ramp so someone can stay in their home, or as comprehensive as teaching someone to navigate every aspect of daily life.

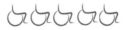

I was first introduced to the independent-living paradigm when I came to Roberts; as mentioned in chapter nineteen, the ultimate goal of the Roberts program is for residents to move to mainstream housing—a standard dorm, an apartment. So, basically, I was there to learn independent-living skills: directing my own personal care, using adaptive equipment, and managing my personal affairs, e.g., finances.

From day one, it was drilled into my head that moving out, and living on my own, was the ultimate golden ticket. I was told it was a chance to radically improve my life, to have the kind of freedom and self-determination as anyone else, etc. etc.

It didn't take long to convince me. The idea that some-one, like me, could live on their own, outside of an assist-ed-living program like Roberts, sounded incredible.

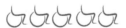

I was all-in on this independent-living thing, and made every effort to prepare myself. I stayed as organized as possible, keeping an absurdly detailed calendar. I also tried my best to maintain a professional relationship with my PAs. I even began to research home-modification equipment, like: an automatic door opener and a portable ramp.

As I honed all of the necessary skills, I started to have this vision of what my future could be: having my own place, commuting to work every day, coming home to my dog—who was happy to see me. It was the dream, and it was within my grasp.

Everyone and everything, in my life, was telling me that living independently was the best thing to do, and I "drank the Kool-Aid," as the kids say.

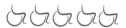

Recall from chapter eighteen that I often refused to accept my limitations, and would put myself in dangerous situations to try and fight them, e.g., refusing to quit math, being carried up the stairs to go to a party.

It always followed the same pattern: I would encounter some new obstacle, refuse to accept it, and try to resist. Then, things would inevitably go wrong, and I would give in, realizing it wasn't worth the trouble.

The move-out situation was more of the same—another losing battle. Only, this time, I was absolutely not willing to give in. Living independently was too important to me; I was going to fight to the bitter end.

It was a hill I was willing to die on—and, as it turned out, I very nearly did.

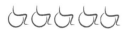

As for how to avoid another situation like that, the answer was two-fold. I had to, first, accept that being completely independent was beyond my reach, that an assisted-living environment was the ceiling for me. And, more importantly, I had to start being realistic with my disability.

Some limitations could not be overcome, no matter how hard I fought. There were some things I just couldn't do, and I had to learn to live with that.

Right then and there, I made a promise to myself: to take every new disability-related obstacle more seriously. Instead of ignoring it, I would look for a solution; I would find a way to accommodate the issue, rather than push back.

CHAPTER TWENTY-TWO

THE INEVITABLE HAPPENS

PART ONE: AN UNWELCOME DEBUT

One night, in early February, we—Alan, Ron, and I—decided to stay up all night. The three of us spent all of our weekly dining hall credits on junk food, watched *Space Jam*, and played *Super Smash Brothers*. It was a great time, the kind of fun only kids can have.

Then, at about six, we decided to get breakfast to celebrate our "accomplishment." I was quite satisfied with myself: "I pulled another all-nighter!" I was feeling pretty good—until we were on the way back.

About three or four blocks from the dorm, I started to feel extremely out of breath. And this wasn't a momentary "let me catch my breath really quick" sort of feeling either; this was much more persistent, and uncomfortable—the air felt heavy, like I was getting into a hot car. I didn't know what was going on, but it wasn't good.

I hurried back to the dorm, and immediately found the floater: "Can you (loud breath) ...help (loud breath) ... me (loud breath)?" He saw how much I was hurting, and ran over: "What's wrong?!" "I need (louder breath) ... the BiPAP mask (louder breath)[40] ... right now (louder breath)!"

---

40 A device for sleep apnea. It helps the wearer breathe by increasing the

He nervously fumbled with the mask, but still managed to quickly get the thing strapped to my face. I took a deep breath, and instantly felt better, letting out a huge sigh of relief.

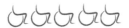

I initially thought the breathing incident was a one-time thing, simply a result of staying up too late. But, over the next week, it happened several more times.

I was sitting in speech class, and, halfway through the ninety-minute lecture, I found it increasingly difficult to pay attention. I was breathing heavy, and felt like I wasn't getting enough air.

I just wanted class to be over, and began watching the clock, counting the minutes until the bell rang. My discomfort continued to escalate, until it became too much; I ended up excusing myself early, and rushing home to put the BiPAP on.

Later in the week, I was out to dinner at Grill Top. It was a make-your-own-stir-fry place, and I piled my bowl high— white rice, Filipino sausage, green peppers, tomatoes, carrots. I gobbled up half of the bowl, gorging until I was completely stuffed.

Then, as I was ready to lean back and enjoy the food coma, it happened again. I started having a hard time

---

air pressure.

breathing, as if my expanded stomach was crushing my lungs.

I was literally panting; I had to get out of there—there was no time to wait for the check. I ended up just leaving my money on the table, and, again, rushing home to put the BiPAP on.

I was at a loss. I had no idea what was going on: "Are these three incidents related?" "Am I fighting a cold?" "Am I not positioned well in my wheelchair?"[41] I was racking my brain, trying to figure out the cause—all the while, hoping it was not a new health problem making its very unwelcome debut.

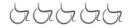

THE INEVITABLE HAPPENS

PART TWO: TROUBLESHOOTING

Unfortunately, these incidents did not stop, and it became clear I had another new symptom to deal with. These were never fun, but they weren't exactly unfamiliar either.

I had played this game many times before; the only difference, this time, was my attitude. I had recently gotten more serious about managing my disability—see the end of the previous chapter—and I wasn't going to ignore

---

41 For wheelchair users, poor seating can cause breathing difficulties.

this new development, or try to fight it. I was going to acknowledge the problem, and find a solution.

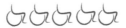

The first step was to find out what I was dealing with, to understand how my breathing issues "behaved." I needed to know: what made the situation worse, what made it better, what triggered it, etc. And, there was only one way to find out.

I began experimenting right away. My first thought was: "This whole thing started when I stayed up all night. Maybe a lack of sleep is the main trigger." So, I started making an effort to go to bed earlier. But no effect—I still had episodes of breathing difficulty. Then, I thought: "Maybe I shouldn't eat to the point of being stuffed. I think it prevents my chest from expanding." So, I began making sure to stop as soon as I was full. But still no effect.

It was slow going at first—I was basically just stabbing around in the dark. But I refused to give up. I continued to investigate, knowing it was only a matter of time before I made a breakthrough.

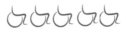

After many more failures, I finally figured it out; I realized why I couldn't find a solution: there wasn't one. My breathing difficulties couldn't be stopped. They weren't in the same category as cavities or obesity, which *can* easily be prevented—brushing your teeth and eating right. My situation was more in the category of diabetes and high blood pressure: a chronic problem that needed to be managed on a daily basis.

In my case, it was all about maintaining my energy level, and avoiding exhaustion. I could only breathe on my own, without the BiPAP, for so long; my chest muscles would eventually get tired. If I went any longer than two or three hours, I would start to feel out of breath.

After I understood this, the answer was simple. All I had to do was wear the BiPAP a few extra times throughout the day. I would wear the mask, for a few minutes, every two hours or so—giving my chest muscles a rest, and staving off exhaustion.

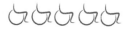

THE INEVITABLE HAPPENS

PART THREE: MIGHT AS WELL MASK

Right away, I noticed a huge difference: I was breathing better, could focus more, and had more stamina. "Man! How bad was I breathing before? Because I can't believe how much better I feel with the BiPAP on!"

I felt so good, in fact, I looked for more opportunities to wear the BiPAP: "What about during my free time? Will it make a big difference if my face is obstructed while I'm watching TV? Or just hanging out in the dorm?" I decided it would not, and proceeded with the mask-wearing.

When Alan and Ron came to my room to watch the game, I was wearing the BiPAP; they could barely hear my muffled voice over the TV: "What did you say?" "I didn't catch all of that." I had to repeat myself over and over, but I didn't mind.

Later, when the Roberts crew was having a few drinks, in my room, I, again, chose to wear the mask. I couldn't partake in the festivities, but it didn't bother me. I didn't need alcohol; my drug of choice was oxygen, and I was getting plenty of it.

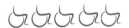

I got so used to the BiPAP that it became uncomfortable to be without it; I began wearing it whenever I got the chance, looking for any reason to mask up—no opportunity was too small, or impractical. Waiting ten minutes for my PA to arrive? Mask. Dictating a paper to my educational assistant (EA)?[42] Mask. Doing anything other than eating or showering? Might as well mask.

Things continued like this until I was eventually wearing the BiPAP all day long.

---

42 Similar to a PA, but, instead of personal care, they help with academic needs, e.g., going to class, doing homework.

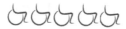

I was barely leaving my room, only venturing out to go to class. And even then, I would hurry home and immediately mask up again.

Now, instead of looking for reasons to *wear* the BiPAP, I was questioning my reasons *not to* wear it: "There are only a few people hanging out in the hall. Is it really worth going out there?" "Some people are going out to the bars tonight. Maybe I should go... Nah, it's not that big of a group." Even when friends actively tried to convince me to come out, I would still have an excuse.

Part of me knew it was not a healthy situation: I was spending too much time by myself, barely socializing outside of my PA shifts. But, a bigger part of me really liked not feeling out of breath constantly. So, I didn't see a reason to change things.

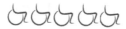

THE INEVITABLE HAPPENS

PART FOUR: THE BARCRAWL

For the first few weeks, my self-imposed isolation wasn't so bad; I didn't feel like I was missing too much. Then, slowly, the lack of friends and fun started to wear on me.

I constantly felt left out: I would see pictures, on Facebook, of events I wasn't a part of; every time I was in the cafeteria, one of my friends would reference something that happened when I wasn't around; and, worst of all, I would be woken up, at two in the morning, by the sweet sound of my drunk friends returning from the bars. It sucked.

After a while, my discipline waned: "Is feeling out of breath really so bad? I mean, it can't kill me." "Is being comfortable worth this? I'm not doing anything. This isn't living!"

I hated feeling trapped, like I couldn't have a life, and started debating with myself whether I should: go out for a night, go to a movie, take a walk, anything.

When the annual Roberts Barcrawl came around, I finally caved. I said to myself: "There's no way I'm missing this!"

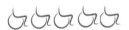

At five hours, the barcrawl would be the longest I was off of the BiPAP in several weeks. If I wasn't careful, I could be severely out of breath by the end of the night. I needed to be prepared.

I meticulously planned every detail, and, by the big night, I was ready: I lied down to rest before the festivities; I made sure to eat earlier, so my stomach wasn't too full;

and, I wore the mask during the pre-game, only joining everyone as they were walking out the door.

I did everything I could, not a second of "breathing-on-my-own" time was wasted. But, despite my best efforts, I still wasn't sure it was enough. I just had to hope for the best.

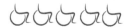

We arrived at the first bar, and I was ecstatic. Fun had recently become a rare occurrence for me, so I wasn't taking anything for granted. I appreciated being with my friends. I appreciated letting loose and having a few drinks. I even appreciated the actual bars themselves.

Everything seemed fresh and exciting again. I was having a blast doing the same old things: having drinks that sounded like candies—lemon drops, gummy bears, Scooby Snacks, mingling with PAs in a social setting, and seeing the confused looks on people's faces, as our giant herd of wheelchairs rolled down the street.

It was great, but, inevitably, that out-of-breath feeling creeped in. It was mild at first—nothing a few drinks couldn't fix—but gradually, over the course of the night, the situation got worse; by the time we were heading to the last bar, I was really struggling.

It would've been wise to head home, but I had my mind set on finishing the crawl.

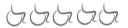

I tried my best to fight through the pain, putting on a fake smile and pretending I wasn't miserable, but it was no use; I couldn't fight it. I soon found myself on the peripherals of the group, panting, barely able to talk.

The situation continued to escalate until it became a full-blown emergency: my chest was burning; I was panting even heavier than before, practically gasping; and I could hear my heartbeat in my ears.

I was in big trouble, and I knew it: "I CAN'T BREATHE! I NEED TO GET TO MY BIPAP!"

I cranked my chair up to full speed, and frantically rushed to the door, aggressively forcing my way through the crowd. I was nearly there when Alan stopped in front of me, drunkenly trying to say something. I yelled—as loud as I could at that point: "Get the hell out of the way!!" and he promptly backed away.

I quickly squeezed out the door, hurrying down the street. From there, it was a frenzied race back to the dorm: riding in the street, zooming through alleys, and practically launching off of curb cuts.

I entered the hallway doors at full speed, praying the floater was not busy. And, luckily, I spotted her in the doorway of another resident's room.

Upon seeing the state I was in, the other resident allowed the floater to help me first. She put the BiPAP mask on me, and it was the most extreme sense of relief I have ever experienced. It was like a drowning person surfacing, and getting that giant gulp of air they had been yearning for.

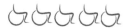

I had plenty of time to think as I sat there, half-drunk, breathing as hard as I could. I realized how dangerous that situation had been: I could have passed out, or worse.

It was certainly scary to consider the possibilities, but fear was not the primary emotion I was feeling; I mostly felt disappointed in myself: "How could I let this happen?" "I thought I was past this sort of thing."

CHAPTER TWENTY-THREE

GETTING MY ACT TOGETHER

In the previous year-and-a-half, I had almost died twice: first with the ulcer, and then nearly suffocating at the barcrawl. Clearly, something needed to change.

It was time to get my act together. And, first on the list was: fixing my breathing situation once and for all.

ᘉᘉᘉᘉᘉ

GETTING MY ACT TOGETHER

PART ONE: BREATHING EASY

I contacted my pulmonologist, and told him what was going on. He said it was probably time to start thinking about permanent ventilation, i.e., a breathing machine.[43]

ᘉᘉᘉᘉᘉ

Growing up, my greatest fear had been being put on a ventilator. The idea of depending on a machine was a

---

43 All people with Duchenne eventually need assisted-breathing.

terrifying prospect; any number of things could go wrong: it could break down, there could be a power outage, someone could press the wrong button and accidentally kill me—I didn't know.

For years, I had completely avoided the idea. I didn't want to hear it from my parents, the doctor, or anyone else. Every time the subject was brought up, I would put up a wall and refuse to listen. And I could have easily responded that way again, but I knew this time was different.

I couldn't avoid it any longer; I needed a ventilator, and that was that. Knowing I had no other choice, I took a deep breath, sighed heavily, and agreed to get one.

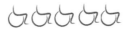

After three weeks of waiting, the ventilator was finally approved by insurance. My respiratory therapist called, and we scheduled a time for him to come set it up for me.

He arrived with two machines, and I was surprised to learn they were both for me: one to sleep with—which would stay in my room, and a portable one to take with me—which would hang on the back of my wheelchair.

I couldn't believe my ears when he told me: "Did you say portable?" "Yes, this one will go with you." "So, it doesn't need to stay in my room?" "No, it has two sets of batteries. The charge lasts about ten hours."

The therapist proceeded to open one of the boxes; as he was pulling out all of the accessories, he asked what kind of mask I used. I showed him my big, ridiculous-looking scuba mask, and he shook his head: "A full-face mask is fine for sleeping, but, during the day, you need something less restrictive."

He pulled a few masks, out of his bag, for me to try. I thought they looked really small, but he explained they were nasal masks—designed to only cover the nose, leaving the face and mouth uncovered.

I tried one, and couldn't believe how much better it was than the "full-face" mask I *had* been using during the day. Not only was it smaller and less cumbersome; I could also talk without my voice being muffled. I could even eat and drink with it. I was pleased to say the least.

It seemed like the good news would never end, but, eventually, the respiratory therapist started wrapping things up: tweaking a few final settings, and giving me his business card.

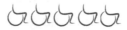

I "rolled out of the shop" with my new vent, and, right away, the improvements were immense. Not only could I breathe more easily; I was breathing better than I *ever* had.

On top of that, I had more stamina. I could jump, from one activity to another to another, without ever needing to rest. I was shocked at how much I could accomplish when I wasn't trapped in my room all the time

ठेठेठेठेठे

My first full day on the vent was jampacked. I went to class *and* participated in discussions *without* panting. I played board games with the guys, *and* could actually be heard: during Monopoly, I was able to argue with Alan when he claimed some b.s. about selling properties to another player.

Then, I went out to dinner with Alan, Ron, and Tom, *and* finished a whole plate of chicken wings *without* worrying about making it until the check. I was even able to stay long after dinner, getting drunk off of fancy cocktails.

The evening continued, until we eventually ended up in Tom's teaching office, having a whiskey, and talking with him into the wee hours of the morning.

It seriously felt like the greatest day of my life. I was able to do what I wanted when I wanted—no need for game-planning, no need to stop and run back to my room every two hours. I was living the good life, and was never going back.

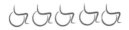

GETTING MY ACT TOGETHER

PART TWO: A PYRAMID SCHEME

Now that my most pressing concern was taken care of, I

could focus on the long-term. I wanted to find some kind of system, or mental framework, to follow that would help prevent future problems, that would help keep my disability under control.

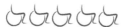

In my psychology classes, I would often hear about a theory called "Maslow's Pyramid." This theory describes how people prioritize their needs. It says that people tend to create a hierarchy of needs, ranking them in order of importance: focusing on the most important first, then the second-most important, and so on.

Specifically, Maslow's Pyramid states that people will address their basic physical needs first—hunger, sleep—before they think about safety—shelter, protection from harm—then comes social needs, and finally accomplishing personal goals.

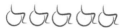

I thought Maslow's Pyramid would make an excellent model for living disabled life. In theory, the hierarchy would make decisions easier. Instead of racking my brain, weighing every option, I would use a simple set of rules to find the best choice.

I would automatically know, for example, not to stay up late to do homework—physical needs over academic ones—or go out to the bars without rearranging my PA schedule first—PA needs over social ones.

I was pretty confident "David's Pyramid" would work, but I had also been burned in the past, so I wasn't making any assumptions until I tried it "in the field."

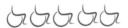

I implemented "David's Pyramid" right away, completely changing my schedule around. And, at first, my new lifestyle was difficult to get used to—with all of the bad habits I had to break—but, pretty soon, I had developed it into a comfortable routine. A typical day looked something like this:

I get up in the morning, finishing my PA shift with time to spare—as usual. But, instead of sending them home early, like I normally would, I make use of the time and do a breathing treatment—I am supposed to do one every morning, but hardly ever do.

Then, instead of watching *The Price is Right* while I wait for the bus, I check my emails and make sure I have everything for class. My educational assistant arrives, and I go to class—*every* class.

I get home, do another breathing treatment, and head to the dining hall. I eat lunch, and, instead of (are you noticing a pattern?) hanging out in the dining hall until my next EA arrives, I lie down and rest for a half-hour. Then,

I work on homework for a few hours, and lie down again until dinner.

After dinner, it's time for my Student Advisory Committee meeting. I am the first one to arrive, and Sharon looks noticeably surprised that I am on time for once.

The meeting adjourns and I hang out, with Alan and Ron, for another hour until my night PA arrives. She gets there promptly at ten—an hour earlier than usual—and I'm in bed before eleven.

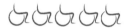

After a few weeks, the new routine was going extremely well. I realized how much confidence one can get from simply handling all of their day-to-day affairs properly. It really gave me a sense of control, over my life, that had been sorely lacking before.

So long story short: the pilot of "David's Pyramid" was a resounding success; I would be adopting it permanently.

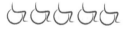

GETTING MY ACT TOGETHER

PART THREE: UNEXPECTED WISDOM

I was happy with every part of my new routine—except

for one. Lying down to rest, multiple times per day, was a boring and tedious chore.

Since I didn't need to sleep, I would just lie awake, staring at the time on my phone. I desperately needed something to occupy my mind.

My solution: reading. I started listening to audiobooks, and, in doing so, came across a book that profoundly changed my life.

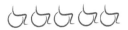

In 1945, Austrian psychiatrist and Holocaust survivor, Viktor Frankl returned home to Vienna. As he reflected, upon his experiences, Frankl became fascinated with the psychology of adversity, and the ways people make sense of difficult situations. This fascination would ultimately lead to the creation of his book: *Man's Search for Meaning*.

The main thesis of the book can be summed up in this passage: "He who has a 'why' to live for can bear with almost any 'how.'" In other words, as long as someone has something meaningful in their life—a personal relationship, a goal, a belief system—they can endure tremendous hardship.

As an example, Frankl describes two of his fellow concentration camp prisoners: one who refused to give up because he had to find his son, and another, a scientist, who kept going because he had to finish his work.

ᑲᑲᑲᑲᑲ

I was really intrigued by this idea of meaning; one passage, in particular, really struck a chord with me: "an individual can still find meaning regardless of their circumstances, even if that meaning is simply to pass through their ordeal with dignity." Upon reading it, I recalled an old memory I had completely forgotten about.

Several years earlier, when I was about thirteen or fourteen, we had taken our yearly trip to Florida to visit my grandpa. And, while we were there, my family had also planned to see my uncle Mitch—my grandpa's brother.

This would be a very important visit because it was the last time we would ever see uncle Mitch. He had terminal cancer, and had maybe a few weeks left.

ᑲᑲᑲᑲᑲ

The day came, and I was honestly expecting it to be a depressing and uncomfortable experience. But, when we got there, it was nothing of the sort. Uncle Mitch was sitting, on the couch, in the living room, just watching TV like nothing was wrong.

We stayed for a few hours, eating lunch and doing some "relative-you-hardly-ever-see" catching-up. And, the entire time, uncle Mitch was in good spirits: laughing, joking, telling stories. I knew he was in a lot of pain, but it didn't show at all.

As we left, I don't remember feeling sad. The only thing I felt was a huge amount of admiration and respect for uncle Mitch. He handled himself with such class, despite everything he had been through, despite knowing it was the end.

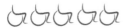

Thinking about my uncle "passing through his ordeal with dignity" inspired me to do the same: "No more feeling sorry for myself." "Complaining just because I have to lie down, twice a day, is not very dignified." "Neither is getting into an emergency where I can barely breathe, and have to rush home." "No more."

From then on, no matter what my disability threw at me, I would face it with dignity. I would try to inspire, in others, the same feelings, of respect and admiration, my uncle Mitch had inspired in me. That would be my "why."

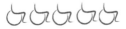

I now had everything I needed to keep my life under control: adequate ventilation, a mental framework to follow, and a healthy sense of meaning when it comes to managing my disability.

From that point forward, my health was always stable and predictable. And, at the time of writing this, it still is.

CHAPTER TWENTY-FOUR

LOOKING FORWARD

I was in a good place now that I finally had my health under control. For the first time in years, my mind was completely clear. I was feeling so good I actually had energy to burn.

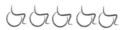

On one of the first nice days of spring, I went for a walk, on the quad, with Alan and Ron. We were mostly shooting the shit, just happy to be outside again after the long winter. There was little conversation, until I broke the silence: "I'm feeling good lately guys. I have all of this energy, and don't know what to do with it."

Ron replied jokingly, "I have a few ideas—" I cut him off, responding indignantly: "Come on man! I'm being serious. I want to start doing something meaningful with my time."

They both could see this was important to me, and stopped teasing. "Okay, so you want to do something meaningful. Like what?" That was a good question. I didn't know.

I continued to ponder the question for the rest of the day. And, that night, my mind was racing with ideas: guest

speaking about disability, creating a list of accessible apart-
ments on campus, making a documentary about Roberts.
The possibilities were endless.

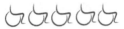

For the next several days, all I could talk about were:
different causes and ideas. It didn't take long for my
enthusiasm to spread to Ron, Alan, and Tom; they quickly
got on board with me, and the four of us met up for a
brainstorming session.

I threw out several ideas to get the conversation
started, but there wasn't much interest until I got to the
documentary.

Ron perked up: "What's that about?" "It would be a
documentary about Roberts, to spread awareness about
the program. We could film ourselves for a year, or maybe
follow a new resident..." Alan interrupted, "Dude! Hell
yeah! Let's do it!"

We were beginning to get excited: "We could be famous!"
"Forget that! We could make a lot of money." "Yeah! We
could get Netflix to buy it! Maybe enter it into some film
festivals!"

Our fantasizing continued, until Tom injected some
reality: "Hold on! Do you guys even know anything about
making movies?" "Well, no. But we can learn." "Ok. Where
are you going to get the money for all of the equipment?"
"Fundraising?" "I think you guys should start small, and

work your way up to a documentary—*if* that's what you really want to do." The three of us let out a collective sigh, and Alan conceded, "You're probably right."

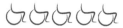

I was feeling deflated after the reality check, and deferred to the group: "You guys got any ideas?" Alan answered, "Nothing specific, but I do like the idea of spreading awareness about Roberts. Maybe we can still do that, just on a smaller scale?"

Again, Tom was the pragmatic one: "I completely agree. But how are we going to do that?" Ron suggested timidly, "A book?" Alan immediately dismissed the idea: "How is that going to work?! There are four of us. Books only have one author, maybe two." Ron pleaded, "Hear me out. I think four authors can work. We would all tell the same story from four different points of view!"

As Ron finished his sentence, the collective light bulb went off. What would allow for telling stories with four different viewpoints? The answer was obvious: a blog!

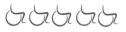

Thus, *The Fine Scholars* blog was born. We each picked a day of the week to post, and got to work.

We proceeded to actually follow through with the plan, and, most surprisingly of all, managed to put out some decent material. Here is a brief excerpt from one of my posts (the quality of writing is much worse than in this book, but, keep in mind, I was ten years younger when these were written):

How much would you say a power wheelchair weighs? If you were to venture a guess, what would it be? 100 lbs? 150? Try 300 lbs! Yep, a power wheelchair will add a good 300 pounds to ya. That means everyone who uses a power wheelchair is technically obese! Bad joke, I know.

Most people mistakenly think power wheelchairs are not heavy. They see how light manuals are—manual chairs are always being folded up, and lifted up stairs, or put in the trunk of a car—and assume the same of power wheelchairs. But trust me, they ain't! Anyone who's ever had their toes ran over by one can attest to that.

I'll often go somewhere with stairs, and someone, one singular person, will say let's just carry it. Me and my dad will look at each other with a devious smirk; to sort of say, "Look at 'Muscles' over here, he's in for a surprise isn't he!" Then when Muscles and 4 other guys actually do lift the chair, its clear they all underestimated the job; sometimes guys will be all red and huffin' and puffin' afterwards. One time I even think I saw some guy limping after.

These things should seriously come with a warning label.

Here is another excerpt. This one should sound familiar, if you recall chapter twenty-one:

Growing up with a disability, you think that different is bad. If I were to try and explain this to someone, without a disability, it would be difficult to convey just how much you want to be like everybody else. For me, the desire was so strong that it influenced a lot of my behaviors—often for the worse.

All throughout elementary school, and even the first two years of high school, I would transfer into a regular desk instead of staying in my wheelchair. My elementary school didn't switch classes, so I would stay in one seat for hours at a time; yep, I chose to limit my mobility even more than it already was, just so I could sit in the same desk as everyone else. Uncomfortable? Oftentimes, yes. Inconvenient? Yes. Unnecessary? Absolutely! And in high school it was the same thing; only this time I had to transfer in and out of my wheelchair for every class. My poor aide had to lift me 12 times a day.

The last thing I wanted to do was admit I was different and give up trying to fight it.

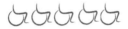

From the very beginning, the blog exceeded all of our expectations: we were getting about twenty or thirty views per day, after just starting, which equated to several hundred views per month; PAs, and other residents alike, were constantly asking when the next post was coming out; and it even opened up some discussions about the topics we were writing about.

We were not only succeeding; we were making an impact. And I was thrilled; I felt like I had found the important cause I was looking for: "Maybe writing is the answer! My ideas have a powerful effect on people!"

I was ready to get serious about blogging, but, without warning, *The Fine Scholars* fell apart. It became clear there were varying levels of interest among the four of us.

Alan and I were posting regularly, but Tom and Ron stopped posting after only a few weeks. This caused a lot of tension, and we started arguing all the time. I eventually said, "Forget it!" and scrapped the whole idea.

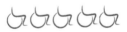

I decided I didn't need to include friends in my "meaningful work," and started looking for a solo pursuit.

I remembered the feeling of satisfaction I got when the

blog was going well, when I saw how my writing affected people, and I wanted that feeling back.

I began to write this book, entirely on my own, and it was exactly what I had been searching for.

CONCLUSION

PART ONE: RECAP

Recall from the introduction that I was reflecting on my accomplishments in college, and had to ask myself: "How did I get here?" The answer to that question was the subject of this book, and I hope you enjoyed reading it. But, before I wrap things up, let's review...

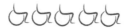

My journey began when I was first diagnosed with muscular dystrophy: learning what having a disability means, and coming to understand how it would affect my life. There were some perks for sure—meeting Jim Carrey with the Make-A-Wish foundation, being unsupervised during recess—but even more challenges. I wasn't able to play sports, I struggled to understand why I was treated differently, and I was forced to confront my grim prognosis.

Then, when things seemed the darkest, I learned about the Roberts program at Generic Midwest University—there actually existed a program that would allow me to go away to college. I applied, got in, and soon found myself living as a resident of the program.

Living at Roberts, I was able to have the "normal"

college experience: I stayed in a dorm, made friends, partied, met girls, and generally had a blast.

I learned to be independent, managing my own life and making my own decisions about my personal care. I also developed socially; my confidence in social interactions improved as I was, for the first time, able to fully relate to my peers—other people with severe disabilities.

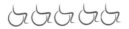

I was breaking through so many barriers, living at Roberts, that I grew to be overconfident: constantly pushing the envelope with my limitations, feeling like I could do anything. And, as a result, I tried to move out of the program.

Of course, that inevitably failed—with no access to around-the-clock assistance, I succumbed to dehydration and exhaustion within a month. This led to a stomach ulcer, and emergency surgery—both of which I was lucky to have survived.

Then, I moved back to Roberts, and thought the difficulties were over. But, shortly after returning, I started to have breathing issues, becoming more-or-less dependent on my BiPAP machine.

I tried my best to manage everything, but was quickly burned out; I grew tired of constantly thinking about breathing, and recklessly decided to go on the entire Roberts Barcrawl.

After literally almost suffocating on the barcrawl, I finally began to approach my health and disability responsibly. I realigned my priorities according to Maslow's Pyramid, and found comfort in the words of Viktor Frankl, author of *Man's Search for Meaning*.

With no more baggage to cloud my mind, I sought out fulfilling ways to spend my time. And, in doing so, I found my passion project: this book.

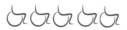

That is about where the journey ends. I went from a clueless kid, completely unaware of how my disability would affect my life, to a well-adjusted, successful adult with a college degree.

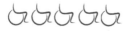

CONCLUSION

PART TWO: PARTING WORDS

I could end this book with some cliché inspirational message along the lines of: "you can do anything you set your mind to," or, "if I did it, you can too," but my readers deserve better.

Instead, let me leave you with this: as impressive as my accomplishments may seem, I didn't do any of it alone. Whether it was my parents doing everything they could to give me the same opportunities as anyone else, neighbors and friends constructing an elevator at my school, or my PAs helping me in college, I always had support and encouragement from others.

All I needed to succeed was the opportunity—that's all anyone with a disability needs. Give us a level playing field, and we will accomplish great things.

THE END

EPILOGUE

At the beginning of this book, I described the small animal-prism figurines my mom would hang from the kitchen window. I was astounded to learn the rainbow-colored light was always present, just hidden from my view.

I was shown something I couldn't see on my own, and I hope this book, in some small way, has done the same for you when it comes to disability. I hope this book has been your prism.

Acknowledgments

- I would first like to thank my mother, who has done the most to help me complete this book. She was the first to read my terrible first draft, and every subsequent draft of the book, giving me honest feedback all the way. She also did all the little things. My mom was there to set me up with my computer and microphone every time I wanted to write, there for every bathroom break, there to suction me every fifteen minutes, there when I stayed up late on my phone making edits, and basically there for anything else.

- I would also like to thank my family as a whole— my mom, dad and sister—for being the only ones who weren't afraid to give me the kind of brutally honest feedback I needed. Without that, my book wouldn't have been nearly as good.

- I would like to thank my editor Eric for his patience and hard work, and for pointing me in the right direction whenever I got lost. He had the unenviable task of reworking my original rough draft, and trying to make sense of it—which he accomplished with flying colors.

- I would like to thank those individuals who typed my edits. I had them working on my tedious and painfully thorough edits for two full years. They also helped with all the other nuts and bolts of publishing—sending emails, managing my Facebook page, signing up for publishing companies, etc.

- I would like to thank John for being my first and only beta reader, as well as my unofficial second editor and creative consultant. He is the one that talked me down from the cliff of completely changing the title, and scrapping several chapters.

- I would like to thank those individuals who gave me permission to write about things that pertain to them, especially with the dating chapter, which contains particularly sensitive material. I'm also grateful to Mrs. Edgerley for allowing me to share details of her son's passing.

- And finally, I would like to thank anyone who was supportive or encouraging to me during this process: Stacy, Nicole, anyone who liked my page on Facebook, and, of course, anyone who reads this book—you are appreciated more than you know.

ABOUT THE AUTHOR

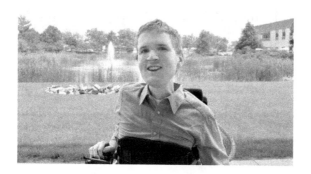

David is currently 30 years old, and lives with his family in Chicago. He grew up in Chicago, and went to the University of Illinois, graduating with degrees in Psychology (B.S. '13) and Social Work (MSW '17). During his time in college, he was able to live on campus, away from home, and be fully independent, thanks to a specialized residence program at the University. The unique living situation gave David the opportunity to have many typical experiences that others with Duchenne do not often get to have.

Recognizing the uniqueness of his experiences was the catalyst for writing this book. David realized that his situation was a perfect case study of how much people with Duchenne can accomplish if given adequate support and encouragement.

Prism is David's first book, and hopefully not his last.

Most of his time is spent writing these days, but when he isn't writing, you can find David discussing disability-related topics on his YouTube channel—Ramp It Up, or following the stock market. David also has an insatiable interest in history and archaeology, specifically ancient Egypt and Rome; he is always looking to learn more, and never misses an opportunity to watch a new history show or documentary. And, when he is not doing any of that, you can find David on a video call with his college friends, playing video games, or relaxing and watching anime.

If you would like to follow David, and keep up-to-date with future books, or just want to hear more from him, here are his social media links:

Facebook: www.facebook.com/davidkauthorpage

www.facebook.com/rampitup1

YouTube: www.youtube.com/c/rampitup